Emergency
Care Technician
Curriculum

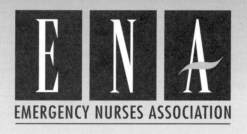

EMERGENCY NURSES ASSOCIATION

JONES AND BARTLETT PUBLISHERS

Sudbury, Massachusetts

BOSTON   TORONTO   LONDON   SINGAPORE

Jones and Bartlett Publishers

World Headquarters
40 Tall Pine Drive
Sudbury, MA 01776
978-443-5000
info@jbpub.com
www.jbpub.com

Jones and Bartlett Publishers
Canada
6339 Ormindale Way
Mississauga, ON L5V 1J2
CANADA

Jones and Bartlett Publishers
International
Barb House, Barb Mews
London W6 7PA
UK

Production Credits
Acquisitions Editor: Penny M. Glynn
Editorial Assistant: Karen Zuck
Production Editor: Anne Spencer
Senior Marketing Manager: Alisha Barry
Manufacturing Buyer: Therese Bräuer
Cover, Design, and Composition: Studio Montage
Printing and Binding: Courier Westford
Cover Printing: Courier Westford

Jones and Bartlett's books and products are available through most bookstores and online booksellers. To contact Jones and Bartlett Publishers directly, call 800-832-0034, fax 978-443-8000, or visit our website at www.jbpub.com.

Substantial discounts on bulk quantities of Jones and Bartlett's publications are available to corporations, professional associations, and other qualified organizations. For details and specific discount information, contact the special sales department at Jones and Bartlett via the above contact information or send an email to specialsales@jbpub.com.

The authors, editors, and publisher have checked with reliable resources to provide information that is complete and accurate. Due to continual evolution of knowledge, treatment modalities, and drug therapies, ENA cannot warranty that the information, in every aspect, is current. ENA is not responsible for any errors, omissions, or for the results obtained from use of such information. Please check with your health care institution regarding applicable policies.

ISBN-13: 978-0-7637-1913-5
ISBN-10: 0-7637-1913-7

Library of Congress Cataloging-in-Publication Data

Massey, Donna.
  Emergency care technician curriculum / by Donna Massey and Andrea Novak.
      p. ; cm.
Includes bibliographical references and index.
  ISBN 0-7637-1913-7 (alk. paper)
  1. Emergency medical technicians.
  [DNLM: 1. Emergency Medical Technicians. 2. Emergency Medical Services. W 21.5 M416e 2002] I. Novak, Andrea. II. Title.
  RC86.7 .M383 2002
  616.02'5--dc21
6048   2001050795

Printed in the United States of America
11 10 09 08 07   10 9 8 7 6 5 4 3

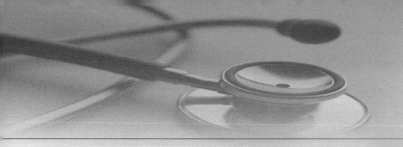

Brief Contents

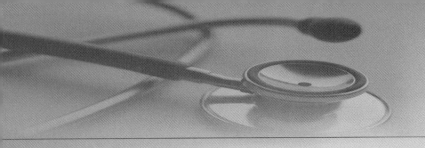

Contents

Preface

This textbook is designed for the high school graduate who is seeking an entry level position into the healthcare field. It is intended to be used as a guide for training healthcare employees in patient care in the emergency department setting, and assumes a basic understanding of the body and its functions. To assist the reader, medical terms that might be unfamiliar are highlighted in bold and defined in the glossary at the end of the book. In addition, frequently used medical abbreviations are readily accessed on page 143.

Acknowledgements

The Emergency Nurses Association (ENA) would like to extend its appreciation to the Emergency Technician Work Group for the development and implementation of the Emergency Technician (ET).

Editors

Kelly A. Hubbell, RN, CEN
Nurse Educator, Emergency Department
UCLA Medical Center
Los Angeles, CA

Andrea Novak, RN, C, MS, CEN
Associate Director of Education
Southern Regional Area Health
Education Center
Fayetteville, NC

Emergency Technician Work Group

Shelly Cohen, RN, BS, CEN
Educator/Consultant
Health Resources Unlimited
Springfield, TN

Ellen M. Johnson, RN
Clinical Instructor/Staff Nurse
Emergency Department
St. Paul Ramsey Medical Center
St. Paul, MN

Contributing Authors

Bonnie L. Baird, RN, MN, CCRN CN III
Critical Care Transport Nurse
University of California, Los Angeles
Los Angeles, CA

Jeff Berg, RN
Cardiac Telemetry Staff Nurse
Rockford Memorial Hospital
Rockford, IL

Vicki Cadwell, RN, MS, CEN, CCRN, MICN
Clinical Educator, Emergency Services
St. Jude Medical Center
Fullerton, CA

Pamela J. Ewald, RN, CEN, MICN
Registered Nurse
UCLA Medical Center
Emergency Medicine Center
Los Angeles, CA

Cathy Jackson-Bruce, RN, BSN
Clinical Educator
Emergency Department
OSF Saint Francis Medical Center
Peoria, IL

Zeb Koran, RN, CEN
Director, Board of Certification
Emergency Nurses Association
Des Plaines, IL

Claudia Niersbach, RN, JD, CEN
Assistant Corporation Council
Department of Law, Torts Division
City of Chicago
Chicago, IL

Anne Scott, RN, CEN, MICN
Pre-hospital Care Coordinator
St. Jude Medical Center
Fullerton, CA

Marcia Bubash Santini, RN, CEN, MICN
Staff Nurse, Emergency Medical
Department
Clinical Instructor, Pre-hospital Care
UCLA Medical Center
Los Angeles, CA

Content Reviewers

Donna Massey, RN, MSN
Associate Director, Educational Services
Emergency Nurses Association
Des Plaines, IL

Sherri-Lynne Almeida, RN, MSN, MEd, DrPH, CEN, EMT-P
Vice President, Client Services
Team Health Southwest
Houston, TX

Patricia Kunz Howard, RN, MSN, CCRN, CEN
Project Director, Delay Trial
UK College of Nursing
Lexington, KY

Staff Liaison

Donna Massey, RN, MSN
Associate Director, Education Services
Emergency Nurses Association
Des Plaines, IL

George Velianoff, RN, DSN, CHE
Interim Executive Director
Emergency Nurses Association
Des Plaines, IL

Chapter 1

The Emergency Technician: Roles and Responsibilities

Introduction

The health care team attends to the physical and emotional needs of patients and their families who come to the emergency department. The ET is a valued member of this team (see **Table 1-1**).

The Role of the Emergency Technician

The ET performs a variety of patient-related duties under the direct supervision of the RN. Hospital policy and procedure will determine the scope of practice in each facility.

Sample tasks the ET may be assigned include the following:

- Clean examination rooms.
- Assemble crutches.
- Assemble equipment.
- Order and restock supplies.
- Collect and transport specimens.
- Assist with admission and discharge of patients.
- Perform clerical tasks.
- Obtain vital signs.
- Document in patient records.
- Clean wounds.
- Bandage and dress wounds.
- Simple splinting of extremities.
- Perform 12-lead electrocardiograms.
- Perform cardiopulmonary resuscitation.
- Remove **sutures**.

The Registered Nurse (RN) is responsible for delegating task assignments. There may be circumstances when another member of the health care team requests assistance. Always ask for explanations and supervision if uncertain about performing a task. The ET is responsible for recognizing if he or she has not received proper training or if the request is beyond his or her scope of practice.

Table 1-1 Members of the Health Care Team

Team Member	Role	Responsibility
Medical Doctor (MD, DO)	• Directs the health care team	• Evaluates patient, determines diagnosis and course of treatment
Registered Nurse (RN)	• Coordinates activities of team members • Licensed by State Board of Nursing	• Directly accountable for patient care • Collaborates with physician to determine priority of care • Delegates tasks
Licensed Vocational Nurse (LVN) or Licensed Practical Nurse (LPN)	• Provides patient care under direction of RN • Licensed by State Board of Nursing	• Performs clinical tasks as defined by the State Nurse Practice Act
Allied Health Providers: • Respiratory Therapists • Social Workers • Medical Technologists • Pharmacists • Radiologic Technologists • Physical and Occupational Therapists	• Works with emergency department team members to assess and intervene with the patient and family member	• Performs specialized services for the patient and family while in the emergency department
Prehospital Providers	• Performs duties under guidelines established by the Medical Director	• Assesses, treats, and transports patients to the emergency department based on established protocols
Physician Assistant (PA)	• Provides patient care under supervision by MD	• Assists physician with patient evaluation, diagnosis and treatment
Nurse Practitioner (NP)	• Provides patient care in collaboration with MD	• Evaluates patient, diagnoses and treats in collaboration with medical doctor and team members

Bibliography

Fiesta, J. (1997). Delegation, downsizing, and liability. *Nursing Management,* 28(12),14.

Shade, B., Rothenburg, M.A., Wertz, E., & Jones, S. (1997). *Mosby's EMT Intermediate Textbook.* St. Louis, MO: Mosby-Year Book.

Zimmerman, P. (1997). Delegating to unlicensed assistive personnel. *Nursing 97,* May,71.

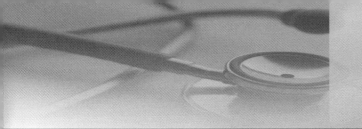

Chapter 2

Communication and Documentation

Upon completion of this module, the learner should be able to do the following:

- List the components of communication.

- Identify three barriers to effective communication.

- Discuss the role body language plays in communication.

- Explain how communication affects public relations.

- Define the purpose of medical record **documentation**.

- Explain two reasons for initiating an incident report.

Introduction

Effective communication techniques are essential in the emergency department. Combining good communication skills with sound customer service results in better patient care, higher patient satisfaction, and decreased stress levels in patients and other health care team members.

Components of Communication

Verbal Communication

Communication involves a message, a sender, and a receiver. For accurate communication to occur, the message sent must be the same as the message received. Components affecting verbal communication include the words used, speech patterns, and tone of voice.

The words of a message must be chosen carefully so that the person receiving the message understands its intent. Factors such as age, socio-economic background, educational background, culture, stress, and illness influence a person's ability to understand messages. Therefore, be very careful about using medical terms when speaking to patients and their families; they may not understand abbreviations such as "NPO" (nothing by mouth), "d/c" (discontinue), or "prn" (as needed).

Patients also may use unfamiliar words when trying to describe their signs and symptoms. A **stroke** may be called a "shock," or fainting may be referred to as "done fell out" in some parts of the country. Speech patterns, including tone, pitch, and speed also affect how well a person understands a message. When under **stress**, a person's speech patterns may speed up or slow down. Speaking too quickly may make it difficult to be understood, while speaking too slowly may result in disinterest or frustration. This is where skill at being able to clarify messages becomes critical. Miscommunication or uncertainty of patient needs can lead to delays in correctly diagnosing and treating a patient. When in doubt, ask the patient to explain further or get help from your other team members to explain the message.

Effective verbal communication includes choosing words that are appropriate, speaking at a normal pace, and using a tone of voice that reflects interest. Verbal communication is only a small component of how a message is received. Nonverbal communication affects a larger percentage of the message.

Nonverbal Communication

<u>Nonverbal communication</u> is conveyed through body language. Examples of body language that affect how the message is being sent include the following:

- Posture
- Eye contact
- Facial expressions
- Physical contact or nearness to others

Entering a patient area with arms crossed, a stiff body posture, and rolling the eyes conveys lack of interest in having meaningful communication. Positive body language includes having a relaxed posture, making eye contact (although some cultures consider direct eye contact rude and aggressive), and showing interest. Positive nonverbal communication will foster trust and encourage sharing essential information needed to assess health care needs.

Touch can be very therapeutic. Appropriate touch reassures most patients that their interests are being addressed and may be calming to the patient. In some situations, however, touch may be perceived as threatening. It may be seen as an invasion of personal space or overstimulation. It takes time and experience to identify situations where touch is appropriate.

Listening is also demonstrated through body language and is an important part of the communication process. Active listening is conveyed by nodding the head, leaning slightly forward, and allowing the other person to speak without interruption.

Barriers to Receiving a Message

Several factors affect how a message is received. Barriers to communication are listed in **Table 2-1**.

Stress

Stress is perceived in the environment by such things as loud noises, unfamiliar surroundings, and smells. Patients and their families may be experiencing internal stress as a result of illness or injury to themselves or to a significant other. People under stress often need information repeated, because stress makes it difficult to concentrate. Speak slowly and use simple terms; avoid using medical terminology. Decreasing the noise level can also reduce stress. Placing a patient or visitor in a quiet environment will help eliminate distractions and decrease stress.

Psychiatric or Emotional Conditions

Communication with psychiatric patients may present a challenge. Some of the techniques listed below can help facilitate effective communication with these patients.

Patients who are depressed may not want to interact with others. Time and patience may help to establish a relationship. It is best to limit the number of people who interact with these patients to prevent overstimulation.

Patients who are **anxious** need frequent reassurance and may not want to be left alone. Explanations must be short, uncomplicated, and repeated, if necessary.

Do not argue with a patient who is mentally disturbed or chemically impaired; arguing only makes a situation worse and could provoke the

Table 2-1 Barriers to Receiving a Message

- Stress
- Psychiatric or emotional conditions
- Age and developmental level
- Cultural differences
- Past experiences
- Privacy and confidentiality issues
- Distractions in the environment

patient to violence. Be polite and calm, yet firm and to the point when communicating. Patients with these impairments do best when limits are set and strictly followed.

Age and Developmental Level

Successful communication must take into account a person's age and developmental level. Toddlers and preschoolers (2–4 years old) need simple, concrete explanations. "Bandage" is easier for a child to understand than "dressing." Use familiar terms for bodily functions. Ask the caregiver what words the child understands when referring to body parts and bodily functions. Be honest when describing how a procedure feels and what will be seen and heard during the procedure. The ability to see or touch equipment may help increase understanding and decrease fears for the younger child.

All children, other than infants, require privacy. Curtains must be drawn during examinations, and body parts kept covered until it is necessary to expose the area. School age children and adolescents do not like to lose control and may feel shame if they cry during a procedure. Therefore, they may need permission to express pain, and their fears.

A child's caregiver has a great impact on the comfort level of the child. __Anxiety__ is contagious. If the caregiver is anxious about what is happening, the child may become anxious as well. Keeping the caregiver informed and involved lessens their fears and helps calm the child.

As people age, it is normal for their hearing and sight to deteriorate. Keep this in mind when communicating with an older individual. Interactions and/or cues from the patient or family often can identify the degree of impairment. When speaking with an older patient with a hearing loss, direct your speech toward the "good" side or make sure the patient can see your lips move as you speak. Slowing down the speech pattern distorts facial movements, making it difficult to be understood. Do not assume that all elderly people are hearing impaired.

Written notes are an acceptable form of communication. Gestures and hand signals can be used to direct the hearing-impaired patient. Patients who use sign language to communicate often bring someone who can interpret for them. Some hospitals also have sign language interpreters on call to facilitate communication with hearing-impaired patients.

Cultural Differences

Today's society is culturally diverse. As a result, people communicate and interpret information in many different ways. Personal opinions regarding individuals from other cultures vary. Each individual possesses certain values and beliefs specific to his or her culture; this makes every individual unique. Consider the following tips when communicating with someone from a different cultural background than your own:

- Speak in a normal tone.
- Be careful of gestures, which can be interpreted differently by different cultural groups.
- Recognize and respect the person's personal space; this may vary with different cultures.
- Be aware of eye contact; direct eye contact in some cultures is very threatening.

Tips for Solving Conflicts:

- Choose a private place for the discussion.
- Describe your impression of the issue or problem.
- Clarify without accusing and without being emotional.
- Restate what has been said.
- Avoid sarcasm, name calling, and insulting comments.
- State your feelings.
- Disagree without being rude.
- Allow the other person to speak without interrupting.
- Be truthful and honest.
- Focus on the issue in question and not on the interpersonal conflict.
- Emphasize the common goals to provide good patient care.
- Get help when needed.
- Know which battles are solvable; there does not have to be a winner and a loser, just a solution.
- Remember that everybody has a bad day and may need understanding.

Another challenge is communicating with a child who speaks English but whose parents do not. Do not ask the child to interpret for a parent except under extreme emergencies and never ask the child to interpret questions of a personal nature. Follow the institution's policy regarding contacting an appropriate interpreter for the patient.

Privacy and Confidentiality Issues

Patients are concerned about their privacy and confidentiality. Curtains must be closed for examinations and during discussions so patients do not feel their personal information is being shared. Communication with family members regarding the patient's condition may be conducted only with the patient's permission. Violating a patient's confidentiality is a serious offense, and many hospitals specify that this is grounds for dismissal.

Handling Conflict

Conflicts may occur in the work environment. Stressful conditions affect communication; however, a stressful environment does not excuse rudeness or inappropriate behavior. Issues should be settled soon after an incident occurs. Personal conflicts must never take priority over patient care.

Responses to stress are learned responses and can be relearned. Be aware of what triggers stress and reactions to stress to control inappropriate remarks or behavior. This is essential to maintain successful communication.

Documentation

Documentation on the patient care record is a means of communication between health care providers. Patient care records are legal documents that provide information on the medical care a patient receives, and the response to treatment. They also serve as evidence in a court of law. Documentation is also used for billing purposes and accreditation issues. Each facility has its own policy governing who is permitted to document in the patient care record. Check with your facility regarding this practice.

Recording Time

There are two methods of recording time: the 12-hour clock which uses a.m. and p.m. and military time, also known as the 24-hour method. Military time begins at midnight, which is referred to as 0000 (zero hundred) hours and 1:00 a.m. is 0100 (zero one hundred) hours. An easy way to remember how to chart using the 24-hour clock is to take the p.m. time and add the number 12. For example, 3:00 p.m. becomes 1500 hours, 4:00 p.m. 1600 hours. Time before 12:00 p.m. is recorded as 0 and then the time. In this case, 8:15 a.m. is recorded as 0815 (see **Figure 2-1**).

Occasionally, despite careful charting practices, a mistake is made. Documentation errors may include writing on the wrong patient chart, or recording incorrect information, times, or treatments. Correct mistakes by drawing a single line through the mistake so that it remains readable, and note above the error that this is a "mistaken entry." Then date, time, and sign above the entry.

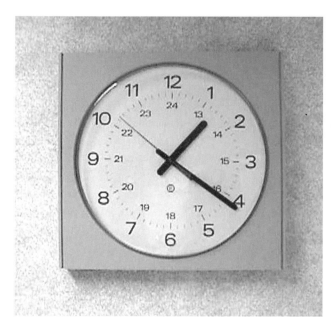

Figure 2-1 24-hour clock.
© ENA

Do's and Don'ts of Documentation

Do

- Write in black ink.
- Write legibly. If the case goes to court, it may be years before you may be asked to testify about what happened, and you will need to be able to read your notes.
- Use correct spelling.
- Use only institution-approved abbreviations.
- Date each new page and time each entry.
- Charting must be to the point, in sequence, and entered when there is a change in a patient's condition or care is given.
- Sign each page with your complete name and credentials, and initial each entry.

Do Not

- Document patient care before it is given.
- Leave blank lines between entries; if needed, draw a line across the blank spaces between entries.
- White out or erase mistakes in charting.
- Scribble over or scratch out what has been written.
- Destroy documentation.
- Argue a point, place blame, criticize, or include personal opinions in a patient's chart.
- Document when an incident report has been filled out on a patient.

Example: 350 ml mistaken entry 5/5/99 9:25 am RM, ET

5/5/99 9:15 a.m.   Assisted patient to bathroom to void. ~~450 ml~~ of clear yellow urine obtained. Patient returned to stretcher.
R. Myers, ET

Another record-keeping problem may occur when information is charted out of sequence or important information is accidentally omitted. In this case, mark what is known as a "late entry." To make a late entry, record the actual time that the entry or note is made. Next, write "late entry from" and the date and time that the entry should have been done. Late entries are useful if they clarify events or conditions regarding patient care.

Example: 7/28/99, 0900. Late entry from 7/27/99, 2300. Patient's belongings given to daughter, C. Jones prior to transport to the operating room.
J. Adams, ET.

Objective and Subjective Documentation

Objective information is what is seen, heard, or measured by individuals other than the patient. Examples include **vital signs**, intake and output, or specific treatments or procedures. It is beyond the scope of practice for the ET to chart subjective information or interpret tests or procedures. Subjective information can be either your own personal bias, judgment, or speculation about the patient such as "drunk," "violent," or "abusive."

It may be appropriate to use subjective statements made by the patient and should always be written with quotation marks around what they say (i.e., "I feel like I have an elephant sitting on my chest" when they are describing chest pain commonly seen with heart attacks).

Incident Report

Incident reports are special records that help examine and identify problems and are considered a form of communication within an institution. An incident report may be filed when there is an error in patient care (i.e., a patient falls out of the bed because the side rails were not raised), patient, visitor, or staff injury, or loss of property.

Most institutions have a Risk Management Department that reviews incident reports. An account of an incident report must never be made on the patient care record, as it is not meant to be part of the patient's legal record.

Patients' Belongings

Patients' personal items can be lost or misplaced in the ED. Identifying and recording a patient's personal items and their location prevents the loss of these items, as well as unnecessary worry for the patient. Remember to obtain the patient's permission and instructions for what to do with his or her belongings. Document in the patient's record the following list of valuables (some hospitals have checklists that are attached to the record):

* Chart general descriptions, yellow or white metal, not gold or silver (i.e., white metal ring with green stone).

* Itemize money in words such as two five-dollar bills.

* Itemize credit cards and personal checks.

* Obtain two employee's signatures to confirm the list of valuables.

* Record the name and relationship of the person to whom you turn over the patient's belongings or valuables.

Customer Service

A customer is anyone who asks for assistance or has a need. Patients, family members, physicians, and coworkers are all customers.

Not everyone is comfortable with the same degree of formality and informality. When speaking to a patient, use his or her full name. It is never appropriate to substitute "honey" or "dear" for the patient's name. Introduce yourself and give your title to inform the patient about your role in his or her care. The patient may give you permission to use his or her first name.

People form an opinion about the ED in a variety of ways. While waiting in the examination room, patients notice whether the room is clean and if the staff behaves in a professional manner. One of the most frequent complaints from patients is long waiting times. A patient or visitor may observe a group of health care providers congregated in one area talking. This may be perceived as a lack of caring by the health care providers as the patient feels their needs are not being met. Check on patients, obtain vital signs, offer blankets, or other comfort measures, and let the patient know what to expect. Patient satisfaction improves when these simple tasks are done on a regular basis.

Summary

Follow the principles of effective communication and understand barriers to communication. Verbal and nonverbal communication and documentation play a role in ensuring that safe patient care is provided.

Bibliography

American Association of Critical Care Nurses. AACN resource for PCA's. *Communication*, 1321.

Booher, D. (1994). *Communicate with confidence! Getting it right the first time and every time.* New York: MacGraw-Hill.

Campinha-Bacote, J., Yahle, T., & Langenkamp, M. (1996). The challenge of cultural diversity for nurse educators. *Journal of Continuing Education in Nursing, 27*(2), 59 64.

Emergency Nurses Association. (1993). Customer relations. In *Orientation to emergency nursing: Diversity in practice.* Park Ridge, IL: Author.

Emergency Nurses Association. (1997). *Approaching diversity: An interactive journey position statement.* Park Ridge, IL: Author.

Emergency Nurses Association. (1998). The pediatric patient. In *Emergency nursing pediatric course (Provider Manual).* (2nd ed., pp. 21–38). Park Ridge, IL: Author.

Hall, J.K. (1996). *Nursing ethics and law.* Philadelphia: Saunders.

Hall, J.M., Stevens, P.E., & Meleis, A.I. (1994). Marginalization: A guiding concept for valuing diversity in nursing knowledge development. *Advances in Nursing Science, 16*(4), 23–41.

Ignatavicus, D., Workman, M., & Mishler, M. (1996). *Medical surgical nursing: A nursing process approach* (Vols. 1–2). Philadelphia: Saunders.

Lipson, J.G., Dibble, S.L., & Minarik, P.A. (1996). *Culture and nursing care: A pocket guide.* San Francisco: Regents, University of California.

Newberry, L. (1998). *Sheehy's emergency nursing: Principles and practice* (2nd ed.). St. Louis, MO: Mosby-Year Book.

Strunk, G. (1996) *The ten commandments of clinical documentation.* Unpublished manuscript.

Chapter 3

Vital Signs

Upon completion of this module, the learner should be able to do the following:

- Identify the normal parameters for pulse, blood pressure, respiratory rate, temperature, and pulse oximetry for the different patient populations seen in the emergency department (ED).

- Select an appropriately sized blood pressure cuff.

- Describe how to obtain orthostatic vital signs.

- State the procedure for applying pulse oximetry.

Introduction

Vital signs refer to the pulse, respiratory rate, blood pressure, and temperature of a patient. Pulse oximetry is considered by many to be a fifth vital sign. The weight of the patient is an additional vital sign in all pediatric patients, and in infants, head circumference. The weight and head circumference give clues to the developmental growth of the infant. Abnormalities of either may indicate additional medical problems. Vital signs are important elements in monitoring the status of the patient and are obtained when the patient is first seen in the ED (usually at triage). They provide a baseline of information for which members of the health care team can track and trend any changes in the patient's condition.

Pulse

The pulse is an indicator of a patient's cardiovascular status. It is felt as a beat where an artery is close to the skin and reflects the pressure of blood against an arterial wall when the heart contracts. Subtle changes in pulse are the first sign of changes in the patient's condition. The pulse is usually counted at the radial artery in a healthy adult. The radial artery is located on the thumb side of the wrist and is felt by pressing the artery with your index and middle fingers. Your thumb must not be used to assess the patient's pulse because the thumb has its own pulse. The pulse beats are counted for one full minute and reported as beats per minute (bpm). The pulse can be taken at other sites if the radial artery is inaccessible or absent, such as the femoral or carotid artery. **Figure 3-1** shows arterial pulse sites.

Note the quality and rhythm of the pulse; it may be fast, slow, irregular, weak or very strong (also called bounding). The rhythm should be regular; however, in children and young adults, the pulse may speed up with inspiration and slow down with expiration. This is a normal condition known as sinus arrhythmia. Ask the patient to hold his or her breath and the irregularity should disappear. Report any irregularity in the pulse to the nurse as it may indicate a serious cardiovascular problem and require placing the patient on a cardiac monitor. If the pulse is difficult to feel (especially in the feet), identify the pulse site with a marker to make it easier to find the pulse the next time it needs to be checked. A Doppler ultrasound device may be used to hear the pulse if it cannot be felt.

The normal pulse rate for an adult ranges from 60 to 100 beats per minute. In the pediatric population, the pulse rate varies with age (see **Table 3-1**). When checking the pulse in children, it is most accurate to listen for the apical (heart) rate with a stethoscope. The brachial artery in the upper arm also may be easily felt in the child or infant.

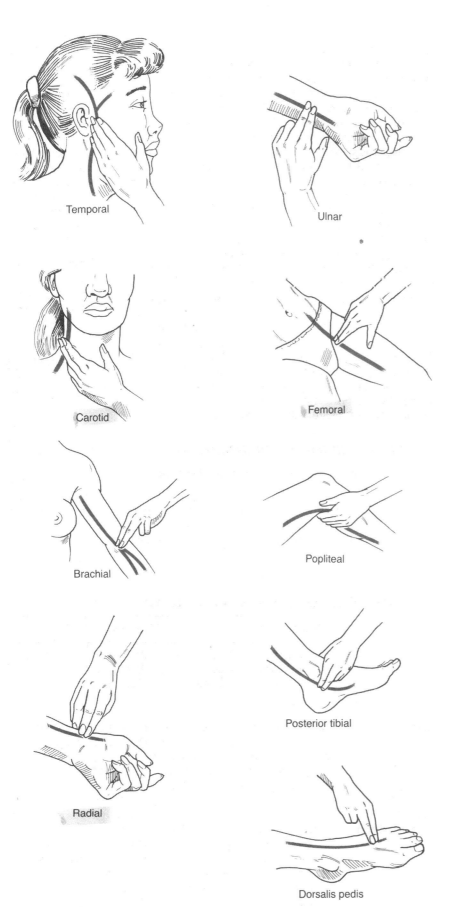

Temporal

Ulnar

Carotid

Femoral

Brachial

Popliteal

Radial

Posterior tibial

Dorsalis pedis

Figure 3-1 Arterial Pulse Sites

(Reprinted with permission from: Dennison, P. D. & Black, J. M. (1993). Nursing care of clients with peripheral vascular disorders. In Black, J. M., & Jacobs, E. M. (Eds.), *Luckmann and Sorensen's Medical-surgical nursing: A Psychophysiologic approach* (4th ed., p. 1263). Philadelphia: Saunders.)

Table 3-1 Pulse, Respiration, and Blood Pressure			
Age	Pulse Beats/Minute	Respirations Breaths/Minute	Blood Pressure (mm Hg)
1 to 28 days	110 to 150	60	80/46
3 months	110 to 140	40	89/60
6 to 12 months	110 to 140	30	89/60
1 year	100 to 140	25	89/60
2 years	90 to 100	20	98/64
3 to 5 years	80 to 100	20	100/70
10 years	70 to 100	15	114/60
Adolescent	70 to 100	12	118/60
Adult	60 to 100	12	120/70

During resuscitation, the femoral and/or carotid arteries are palpated for the pulse. Another method to obtain the pulse is to use a stethoscope and listen for the heartbeat. This is done by placing the stethoscope at the fourth or fifth rib, near the nipple line, on the left side of the chest.

Several conditions affect the pulse rate, such as physical condition, age, medication, fever, fear, or positioning of the patient. Accuracy and an eye for subtle changes with prompt reporting can greatly affect patient outcome. Generally, a pulse below 60 or above 100 beats/minute must be monitored frequently in an adult. Pulse rates that fall below 80 beats/minute in an infant and 60 beats/minute in a child must be reported immediately, as interventions may be required to boost the heart rate (i.e., oxygen, chest compressions).

An increase or decrease in the pulse rate may be the first indication that something is changing in the patient's condition and should be reported and monitored closely.

Blood Pressure

Blood pressure is the force at which the blood surges through the arteries generated by the pumping action of the heart. The blood pressure is measured as a fraction of systole over diastole. Systole reflects the amount of force needed for the heart to contract and push blood into the arteries. Diastole is the resting phase of the heart as it fills with blood from the veins. Blood pressure is measured in millimeters of mercury (mm Hg). An average adult blood pressure ranges from 100 to 140 systolic and 70 to 90 diastolic.

Hypertension (high blood pressure values, such as 160/90 mm Hg or higher) or hypotension (low blood pressure measurement of 90/40 mm Hg or lower) must be reported and a full set of vital signs obtained as well. Many times the patient has additional symptoms, such as headache with hypertension and dizziness with hypotension.

Blood pressure may be affected by pain, stress, medication, exercise, and using the wrong size blood pressure cuff. Too small a cuff gives a false high reading, while a cuff that is too big for the patient gives a false low blood pressure reading.

Electronic blood pressure cuffs are commonly used in the hospital setting. A health care team member must monitor all uses of electronic equipment. The cuff must be wrapped closely around the bare arm and the size of the cuff must be correct for the patient. Placing the cuff somewhere other than the arm (e.g., thigh) must be documented, as these readings will be different than expected. The farther away from the heart, the lower the blood pressure. Electronic monitoring often has a built-in program for adult and pediatric inflation pressures, so it must be set appropriately. Once a blood pressure has been taken, the monitor will inflate the cuff 20 to 30 mm Hg above the previous pressure. Some patients are sensitive to blood pressure monitoring, and an inflation pressure of more than 30 mm Hg above their normal pressure can cause pain, which may affect the blood pressure. Stop the test if it is causing this kind of problem. Some institutions require that the first blood pressure be auscultated (heard with a stethoscope) to ensure accuracy of an electronic monitoring device.

To obtain a blood pressure, use a **sphygmomanometer** with the appropriate size cuff and a stethoscope (see **Figure 3-2**). The width of the cuff should measure two thirds the diameter of the patient's upper arm.

- Place the patient's arm palm up supported on a bed or table.

- Feel for the position of the brachial artery.

- Apply the cuff 1 inch above the elbow with the center of the cuff bladder at the brachial artery.

- Secure the cuff, making sure it is not too tight. The Emergency Technician (ET) must be able to slip two fingers between the cuff and the patient's arm. If the patient is allergic to latex, use a latex free cuff or if one is not available, apply a gauze wrap on the arm before placing the cuff.

- Locate the brachial artery and place the first three fingers over the artery.

- Close the valve attached to the hand pump by turning it clockwise.

- Inflate the cuff 10 mm Hg above the last pulse felt.

- Place the diaphragm of the stethoscope over the brachial artery.

- Slowly deflate the cuff by opening the valve counterclockwise.

- The systolic measurement is the number when the ET first hears the pulse.

- The diastolic measurement is the number when the ET last hears the pulse.

- Document the blood pressure reading in the patient's chart.

Never take a blood pressure in the arm of a patient who has a dialysis shunt in place or an arm that is on the same side as a mastectomy, lumpectomy, or lymph node resection. Avoid taking a blood pressure in the arm with an intravenous line or that is injured, if possible, as it may affect the circulation in that arm.

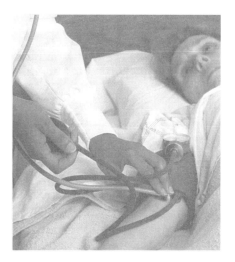

Figure 3-2 Taking a Blood Pressure and BP Machine

(Reprinted with permission from: Hegner, B., and Caldwell, E. (1995). Measuring and recording vital signs, height, and weight. In: *Nursing assistant: A nursing approach* (7th ed., p. 254). Albany, NY: Delmar Publishing.)

Orthostatic Vital Signs

Orthostatic vital signs are used to assess fluid loss caused by factors such as heat, emesis (vomiting), diarrhea, bleeding, or surgery. To obtain orthostatic vital signs, take the blood pressure three times: first while the patient is lying **supine**; second, when sitting upright with legs dangling; and third when standing (if the patient is able to do so). Document these findings by drawing pictures of each part of the orthostatic vital signs and then write the reading next to it.

O———   Patient is lying flat (supine).

Patient is sitting upright.

Patient is standing.

If the patient reports dizziness at any time, stop the evaluation immediately. Allow the patient to return to the stretcher and lie down. A change, such as a drop in blood pressure of 20 mm Hg and/or a rise in pulse rate of 20 beats/minute is considered to be a positive finding. All positive orthostatic vital sign measurements must be communicated to the nurse or physician.

Respirations

Breathing is an automatic function regulated by the medulla in the brain. **Respiration** is the act of breathing. Each breath consists of an **inspiration** and **expiration**. Breathing is normally quiet, effortless, and regular in rhythm. The main function of respiration is to supply the body with oxygen and rid it of carbon dioxide as a waste product. The air we breathe contains 21% oxygen, 78% nitrogen, and the last 1% is chiefly argon. Exhaled air, which really is just a mixture of gases, is 16% oxygen, 80% nitrogen, and 4% carbon dioxide.

Respiratory rate is counted by the rise and fall of the chest for 1 minute. The normal adult respiratory rate is 12 to 20 breaths per minute. The pediatric patient has a faster respiratory rate which varies by age (see **Table 3-1**). Try to count respiratory rate without the patient's knowledge, as he or she may unconsciously change the rate if you are obviously staring at the chest. One way to avoid being obvious is to check the respiratory rate immediately after checking the pulse. The patient will think his or her pulse is still being checked.

When counting the respiratory rate, also note the rhythm, effort (labored), depth (shallow or deep), rise and fall of the chest (equal or **paradoxical** movements), any noise made while breathing, and the color of the skin. Blue tinges (cyanosis) to the lips, tips of ears, and/or tip of the nose or fingers must be reported immediately to the nurse. This is a sign of lack of oxygen to the tissues and cells. Also check the patient for periods of **apnea**, which is the absence of breathing. Count the amount of seconds between breaths in the patient who has apnea.

The effort the patient uses to breathe is very important to assess. Signs of increased effort, such as use of accessory muscles (look at the neck muscles and abdominal muscles for increased work), retractions, or nasal flaring are all abnormal findings and must be reported to the nurse. Infants use their abdominal muscles to breathe so watch the rise and fall of their <u>abdomen</u> instead of their chest wall to count respirations.

Head bobbing, grunting, and high-pitched sounds on inspiration are considered a medical emergency in the pediatric patient. These are signs of airway compromise, and the patient will go into <u>respiratory arrest</u> if not treated appropriately. Adults with noisy respirations may have <u>secretions</u> in the airway and may need to have the passage cleared by suctioning.

Several factors can affect the respiratory rate, such as <u>fever</u>, cold, age, exercise, medication, illegal drugs, illness, and emotion. Each factor is part of the overall clinical picture and must be taken into consideration.

Temperature

Body temperature is the balance of heat production and heat loss. The <u>hypothalamus</u> in the center of the brain controls body temperature. The normal oral temperature range is considered to be between 36.5 to 37.5°C (97.6 to 99.6°F).

There are several types of thermometers: Mercury, electronic, paper, <u>tympanic</u>, and electronic probe. Thermometers may be placed in the mouth, ear, axilla (armpit), or rectum to obtain a body temperature. Oral thermometers must be placed in the pocket of tissue under the tongue against the sublingual artery. Make sure the patient's lips cover the thermometer as well; suggest the patient purse the lips like a kiss and avoid biting down on the thermometer. If the patient has had anything to eat or drink wait at least 15 minutes before taking an oral temperature as this may affect the results. Patients on oxygen or those who breathe through their mouths should have their temperature taken by an alternative method, since the reading will not be accurate. Children younger than 4 years old usually cannot hold an oral thermometer properly in their mouths for the necessary length of time.

Rectal thermometers and probes must be placed next to the rectal wall approximately 3 inches deep for the adult and $\frac{1}{2}$ to 1 inch for the pediatric patient. Hold on to the thermometer to prevent injury to the rectum, especially for children. A patient who has diarrhea or rectal bleeding should not have this form of temperature measurement. Large amounts of stool in the rectum may make it difficult to obtain an accurate reading, because the tendency is to take the temperature of the stool and not the true body temperature. Rectal temperatures register -17.2°C (1°F) higher than temperatures taken with oral thermometers.

Oral thermometers used at the axillary site must be held with the arm closed over the thermometer and next to the body to seal out environmental factors. This is an easy way to check the temperature of a patient who cannot keep the probe safely in his or her mouth, is on oxygen or breathes through their mouth.

The tympanic probe is placed in the ear canal while gently pulling on the ear to straighten the line of site to the <u>tympanic membrane</u>. Do not use the tympanic probe when the patient has an ear infection, large amounts of earwax, injury, or any drainage from that ear.

Precautions must be taken to ensure patient safety and prevent injury. A confused or combative patient should not have his or her temperature taken without precautions, such as additional staff or other interventions by the nurse.

Cooling Measures

Hyperthermia is defined as a core body temperature of greater than 40.5°C (105°F). It is most serious in **neonates** (newborns) and the elderly. It can be caused by infections, exposure to high external temperatures, illegal drugs, medication, and neurologic injuries, such as stroke or head trauma. Symptoms include fever, hot flushed skin, headache, confusion, weakness, loss of energy, tachycardia, tachypnea, and possibly low blood pressure. Death occurs if not treated promptly. Treatment includes rapid cooling by removing the patient's clothing, giving the patient a **tepid** bath, packing the vascular areas with ice padded in the groin, armpits, and the back of the neck, or putting a cooling blanket under the patient. These measures are performed quickly with frequent changes in ice or water to maintain a cool environment. A rectal temperature or continuous rectal probe is used to monitor the effectiveness of treatment.

Warming Measures

Hypothermia is defined as a core body temperature of less than 35.0°C (95.0°F). It can be caused by a prolonged exposure to cold from water or air, by illness, or deliberately induced during surgery. As the body temperature drops to the 32 to 35°C (90 to 95°F) range, associated symptoms such as confusion and shivering can develop. It is impossible to monitor cardiac status in a patient who is shivering. A common problem in the ED is lack of identification of hypothermia in the confused elderly patient or the combative alcoholic patient. As body temperature drops to 30°C (86°F), shivering ceases and profound unconsciousness occurs. At 28°C (82°F), there is a high incidence of **cardiac arrest**. Be sure to use a thermometer that has an appropriate hypothermia range. Treatment focuses on preventing further heat loss. The cold patient must be warmed with the utmost of care. Wet clothes must be removed, the skin dried, and some form of insulation provided. The air temperature must be warm. Heat lamps can help warm the patient. Apply warm blankets on and around the patient and change frequently to maintain warmth. Wrap the head in a warm towel if the hair is wet. The same blanket machine used for the hyperthermic patient can also provide a warming environment. A sleeping bag type blanket is a great help because it can trap the warm air surrounding the patient.

A rectal probe is used to monitor the temperature. Because there is such a profound metabolic and cardiac component to this state, studies have shown that a gradual rise in temperature of 1°C (6.4°F) per hour results in the best patient outcome. The patient must be handled very gently, as there is a high incidence of cardiac arrest with rough handling. The patient also may lose his or her **gag reflex** and be at risk for airway problems. Vital signs are difficult to obtain. It may take as much as 1 to 2 minutes to feel or hear a pulse. For severe hypothermia, the patient is warmed from the inside out. This is done through irrigating the bladder, peritoneum, stomach, and other body parts with warmed fluids.

Pulse Oximetry

Pulse oximetry is a noninvasive method to continuously measure the amount of oxygen in the blood. It is considered by some health care professionals to be the fifth vital sign and is useful for completing a rapid assess-

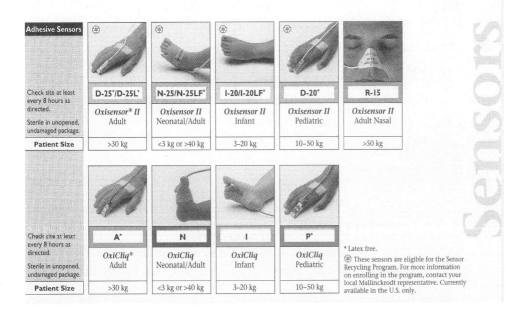

NELLCOR SENSOR SELECTION GUIDE

Adhesive Sensors	**D-25°/D-25L°**	**N-25/N-25LF°**	**I-20/I-20LF°**	**D-20°**	**R-15**
Check site at least every 8 hours as directed.	*Oxisensor® II* Adult	*Oxisensor II* Neonatal/Adult	*Oxisensor II* Infant	*Oxisensor II* Pediatric	*Oxisensor II* Adult Nasal
Sterile in unopened, undamaged package.					
Patient Size	>30 kg	<3 kg or >40 kg	3–20 kg	10–50 kg	>50 kg

Check site at least every 8 hours as directed.	**A°**	**N**	**I**	**P°**
Sterile in unopened, undamaged package.	*OxiCliq®* Adult	*OxiCliq* Neonatal/Adult	*OxiCliq* Infant	*OxiCliq* Pediatric
Patient Size	>30 kg	<3 kg or >40 kg	3–20 kg	10–50 kg

* Latex free.

⊛ These sensors are eligible for the Sensor Recycling Program. For more information on enrolling in the program, contact your local Mallinckrodt representative. Currently available in the U.S. only.

Figure 3-3 Pulse Oximeter and Selection of Probes Attached to Different Body Sites

(Reprinted with permission from Mallinckrodt, Inc., St. Louis.)

ment of patient status, response to treatment, and to assess the severity of the illness. A sensor is attached to part of the body (e.g., finger, toe, infant heel, earlobe, nose—see **Figure 3-3**). Remove nail polish before applying the probe as it may interfere with the reading. A normal pulse oximetry reading in an adult ranges from 95 to 100% saturation. Adults with chronic obstructive pulmonary disease (COPD), such as **emphysema** or **asthma**, typically have a lower saturation level. An oxygen saturation level of less than 70% is considered life-threatening.

Certain conditions affect the accuracy of the reading. Carbon monoxide poisoning, low **perfusion**, **edema**, movement, **anemia**, and hypothermia give false readings.

The pulse oximeter has alarms that may be set for long-term monitoring of the patient.

Summary

Vital signs are important indicators of the health status of the patient. Accurate measurement, trending, and tracking of vital signs will alert the Emergency Technician of early changes in the patient's condition. Early recognition of changes can lead to early intervention, resulting in better outcomes for the patient in the ED.

Bibliography

Elixson, E.M. (1991). Hypothermia: Cold-water drowning. *Critical Care Nursing Clinics of North America,* 3(2), 287-292.

Groer, K. (1989). *Physiology and pathophysiology of the body fluids.* St. Louis, MO: Mosby-Year Book.

Hegner, B., & Caldwell, E. (1995). *Nursing assistant: A nursing process approach* (7th ed.). Albany, NY: Delmar.

Newberry, L. (1998). *Sheehy's emergency nursing: Principles and practice* (2nd ed.). St. Louis, MO: Mosby-Year Book.

Upon completion of this module, the learner should be able to do the following:

- Identify the role of the Emergency Technician (ET) in caring for the patient with a respiratory emergency.

- Explain the procedure for obtaining a peak flow.

Respiratory System

Introduction

Airway and breathing must be evaluated and treated for all emergency department (ED) patients before any other interventions are considered. Respiratory emergencies can occur from chronic conditions, such as emphysema, or from acute conditions, such as <u>hemothorax</u> or an <u>anaphylactic</u> reaction.

Anatomy and Physiology

The pulmonary (respiratory) system is made up of those organs and structures that assist in breathing or the process of oxygen delivery. The pulmonary system is divided into the upper and lower respiratory tracts (see **Figure 4-1**). The upper respiratory tract includes the nose, pharynx (throat), larynx (voice box), and trachea (windpipe); the lower respiratory tract includes the trachea, bronchi, and lungs (see **Table 4-1**). The upper respiratory tract is located outside of the thoracic cage (chest), and the lower respiratory tract is located almost entirely within the thoracic cage.

Breathing Terminology

- Ventilation is the process that moves air into and out of the lungs.

- Respiration is the physical and chemical process by which an organism supplies its tissues and cells with the oxygen needed to live.

- <u>Inspiration</u> is the process of taking air into the lungs.

- <u>Expiration</u> is the process of moving air out of the lungs (see Figure 4-2).

Pediatric Respiratory Considerations

Many of the patients with respiratory problems treated in the ED are infants and children. The respiratory system for this special patient population is slightly different than that of the adult.

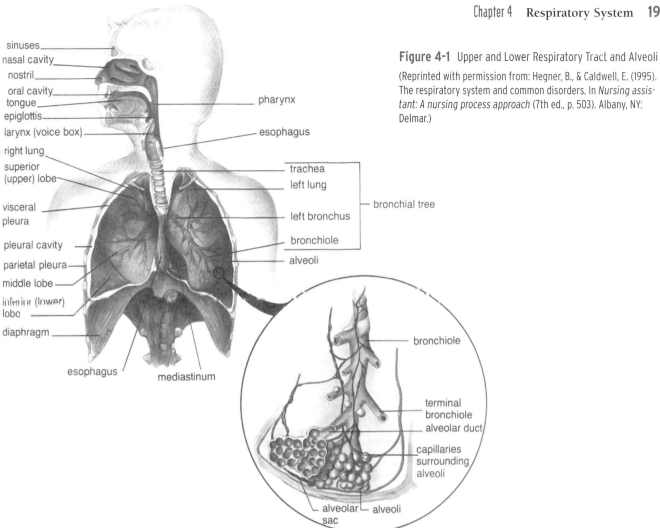

Figure 4-1 Upper and Lower Respiratory Tract and Alveoli
(Reprinted with permission from: Hegner, B., & Caldwell, E. (1995). The respiratory system and common disorders. In *Nursing assistant: A nursing process approach* (7th ed., p. 503). Albany, NY: Delmar.)

Table 4-1 Upper and Lower Respiratory Tracts	
Structure	**Function**
Upper Respiratory Tract	
Nose	Filters, warms, and humidifies inhaled air
Pharynx	Serves as passage for air to the lungs and food to the stomach
Larynx	Includes the vocal cords (voice box)
Epiglottis (Flap)	Prevents food from going into the lungs
Esophagus	Passes food through to the stomach
Trachea	Moves air into the lungs and lower respiratory tract
Lower Respiratory Tract	
Lungs	Organ of respiration that houses the lower respiratory tract
Bronchus	Splits off trachea into two tubes to bring air into lung fields
Bronchioles	Brings inhaled air to alveoli
Alveoli	Permits gas exchange between lungs and blood

Figure 4-2 Inspiration and Expiration

(Reprinted with permission from: Atrium Medical Corporation. (1999). *Managing chest drainage* (p. 26). Hudson, NH: Author.)

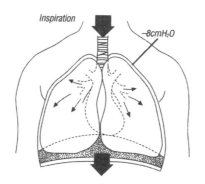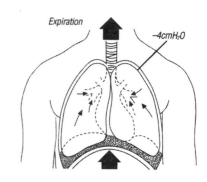

Tips to care for respiratory problems in the child and infant:

- Infants are strictly nose breathers through the first months of life. **Patency** of the nose and pharynx are essential. Be sure a bulb syringe is available (see **Figure 4-3**).

- The tongue is larger. A tongue blade may be used to help insert an oral airway.

- The larynx is higher and narrower in diameter. Uncuffed endotracheal tubes (up to age 8) are used in infants and children (see **Figure 4-4**).

- The trachea is easily obstructed by flexion or hyperextension. Keep the head in a neutral (sniffing) position (see **Figure 4-5**).

- Infants have twice the oxygen requirements of adults because of their rapid growth. Oxygen may be delivered by additional means such as "blow by" (see **Figure 4-6**).

- Children younger than age 7 have immature and weak accessory muscles. They tire more easily when their airway is compromised. There is increased **compliance** of the rib cage, resulting in **retractions**. Be sure to have oxygen readily available.

- Children younger than age 3 and up to age 7 years are primarily abdominal breathers. Watch for rise and fall of the abdomen to count respiratory rate.

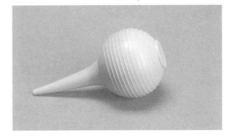

Figure 4-3 Bulb Syringe

(Reproduced with permission from: American Academy of Pediatrics. (2000). Oxygen delivery. In *Pediatric education for prehospital professionals* (p. 241). Elk Grove, IL: Author.)

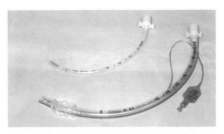

Figure 4-4 Cuffed versus Uncuffed ET Tube

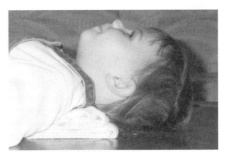

Figure 4-5 Child in the Sniffing Position

(Photographed by Donna Massey, RN, MSN.)

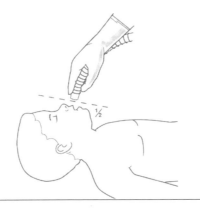

Figure 4-6 "Blow by" Oxygen

(Reprinted with permission from: French, J.P. (1995). Oxygenation and ventilation. In *Pediatric emergency skills* (p. 80). St. Louis, MO: Mosby-Year Book.)

Respiratory Disorders

Disorders of the respiratory system result from a variety of causes, including obstruction, spasm, or pressure (see **Table 4-2**). An example of obstruction is food that enters the larynx instead of the esophagus. If the food completely blocks the larynx, air is unable to pass into the lungs. An example of spasm is asthma, in which the airway spasms as a result of an irritant. This spasm decreases the ability to provide oxygen to the blood. A tension pneumothorax is an example of a pressure problem. A tension pneumothorax is caused by trauma to the chest wall. Air enters the pleural space and exerts pressure against the lung. As the pressure increases the lung collapses, decreasing the ability to deliver oxygen to the blood. Left untreated, the patient will die.

Table 4-2 Respiratory Disorders

Disorder	Condition or Result
Airway Obstruction	The blocking of some part of the airway by an object or spasm preventing it from functioning normally
Asthma	Chronic inflammatory disorder of lower airway that causes spasm. Spasm and mucus plugging decreases the ability to oxygenate the blood
Chronic Obstructive Pulmonary Disease (COPD)	Destruction of the walls of the alveoli, resulting in fewer alveoli to deliver oxygen to the blood. Emphysema is a type of COPD.
Flail Chest	When two or more adjacent ribs are broken in more than two places on the same rib, causing that area of the thoracic cage to become unstable
Hemothorax	Blood in the pleural space (see **Figure 4-7**)
Pneumohemothorax	Blood and air in the pleural space
Pneumonia	Inflammation of the lungs caused by bacteria, viruses, or chemical irritants
Pneumothorax	Air in the pleural space (see **Figure 4-7**)
Pulmonary Edema	Fluid in the alveoli and tissues of the lungs
Pulmonary Embolism	A blood clot in a pulmonary artery that prevents a portion of the lung from exchanging gases
Tension Pneumothorax	Air in the pleural space that is under pressure caused by trauma

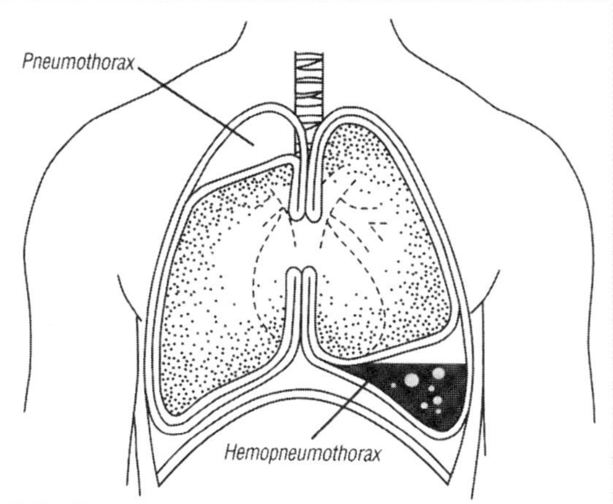

Figure 4-7 Pneumothorax and Hemothorax

(Reprinted with permission from: Atrium Medical Corporation. (1999). *Managing chest drainage* (p. 27). Hudson, NH: Author.)

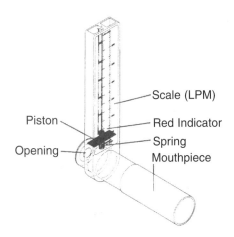

Figure 4-8 Peak Expiratory Flow Meter

(Reprinted with permission from: Respironics Health Scan Asthma & Allergy Products. Cedar Grove, N.J. 07009, 2001.)

Peak Expiratory Flow Rate

A peak expiratory flow rate (PEFR) is often obtained from patients with asthma to measure the flow rate during a maximum expiration (i.e., The patient blows hard, as if they are blowing out candles (see **Figure 4-8**). It is measured in liters per minute (L/m) and is used to measure the severity of the asthma as well as monitor the patient's response to therapy. The more severe the asthma attack, the lower the PEFR reading. Remember to reset the needle on the meter back to zero before the next PEFR is measured.

Normal values are related to the patient's height as follows:

Height (cm)	PEFR (L/min)
120	215
130	260
140	300
150	350
160	400
170	450
180	500

The PEFR is obtained by using a Wright meter. A disposable mouthpiece is placed into the meter. The patient is instructed to take a very deep breath and then exhale as hard as he or she can into the meter. Repeat the PEFR twice and record the highest reading.

Oxygen Therapy

Oxygen therapy is used for many different reasons: To treat **hypoxia**; to decrease the workload on the heart; and to decrease the work of breathing. It is important to remember that oxygen is considered a medication and cannot be independently initiated by the ET.

In the ED, wall outlets are available to attach the oxygen delivery devices. While transporting patients, a portable oxygen cylinder is used. A flowmeter is connected to the pressure regulator (or directly into the wall in the ED) to control the flow of oxygen in liters per minute. This usually ranges from 0 to 15 L/min. The oxygen delivery device is connected to the flowmeter to deliver oxygen to the patient (see **Figure 4-9**).

Figure 4-9 A. Close-up View of Regulator and Ball-type Flowmeter. **B.** Close-up View of Regulator and Needle-gauge Flowmeter

(Reprinted with permission from: Slabach, R. (1999). Application and removal of oxygen tank regulators. In Proehl, J. A. (Ed.). *Emergency nursing procedures* (2nd ed., pp. 80-81). Philadelphia: WB Saunders.)

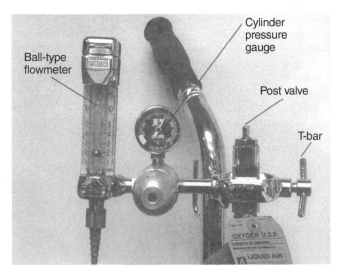

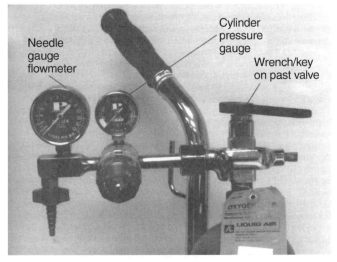

Oxygen Adjuncts

Several different devices can deliver oxygen to patients. It is important to become familiar with these devices to properly apply them on the patient.

Nasal cannula: A commonly used oxygen delivery device used on patients who are breathing spontaneously. Flow rate should not exceed 6 liters per minute, which delivers up to 45% oxygen. The actual amount of inspired oxygen depends on the patient's respiratory rate and depth. This type of device is well tolerated by most patients (see **Figure 4-10**).

Face mask: The face mask may also be used on patients breathing spontaneously. Air holes on the sides of the mask allow passage of inspired and expired air. Recommended flow rate is 5 to 10 L/m, which provides 40 to 60% oxygen. Most patients can tolerate the face mask, except those with severe <u>dyspnea</u> (see **Figure 4-11**).

Partial rebreather mask: A face mask is attached to a reservoir bag, allowing patients to inhale oxygen-rich air from the bag.

Nonrebreather mask: Similar to the partial rebreather mask, this mask has two valves between the mask and reservoir bag. The mask must fit snugly on the patient's face to prevent room air from mixing with the oxygen in the reservoir bag. One valve prevents exhaled air from entering the bag, and the other valve allows gas to leave the mask during exhalation, preventing room air from entering during inspiration. Carbon dioxide can accumulate if the reservoir bag is pinched or there is obstruction in the inhalation valve. The patient inhales 100% oxygen from the properly inflated reservoir when the flow rate is set at 12 to 15 L/m (see **Figure 4-12**).

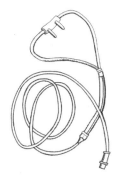

Figure 4-10 Nasal Cannula

(Reprinted with permission from: Slabach, R.. (1999). General principles of oxygen therapy and oxygen delivery devices. In Proehl, J.A. (Ed.). *Emergency nursing procedures* (2nd ed., p. 76). Philadelphia: WB Saunders.)

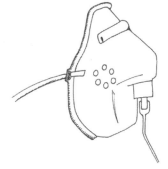

Figure 4-11 Simple Face Mask

(Reprinted with permission from: Slabach, R. (1999). General principles of oxygen therapy and oxygen delivery devices. In Proehl, J.A. (Ed.). *Emergency nursing procedures* (2nd ed., p. 76). Philadelphia: Saunders.)

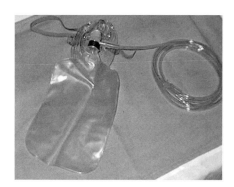

Figure 4-12 Nonrebreather Mask

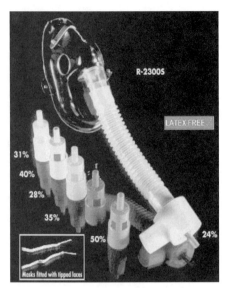

Figure 4-13 Venturi Mask
RESPAN Products, Inc; Ontario, Canada.

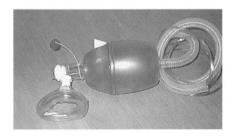

Figure 4-14 Bag-Valve-Mask

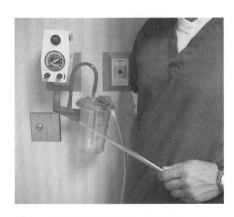

Figure 4-15 Wall Suction with Tubing and
Tonsil-Tipped Suction Attached

Venturi mask: This mask is used for patients who have a history of chronic obstructive pulmonary disease or experiencing **respiratory distress**. It allows the delivery of a fixed concentration of oxygen. Patients may find this type of mask uncomfortable with prolonged use (see **Figure 4-13**).

Pocket mask: This mask is used for mouth-to-mask artificial ventilations, which avoids contact with the patient's mouth. Be sure the mask covers the nose and mouth. Tilt the patient's head back, using the jaw thrust or chin lift maneuver and blow directly into the tube on the top of the mask.

The air you breathe into the pocket mask will provide the patient with approximately 16% oxygen. (Room air contains 21% oxygen)

Bag-valve-mask: (BVM) This device includes a face mask, a self-inflating bag, and a nonrebreathing valve (see **Figure 4-14**). Apply this mask the same way as the pocket mask. Be sure the mask is sealed around the nose and mouth. An oropharyngeal or nasopharyngeal airway may be used in conjunction with the bag-valve-mask. The bag without the mask may be used to assist ventilations with an endotracheal tube.

A BVM with a reservoir attached will deliver 90 to 100% oxygen at 12 to 15 L/m. This device, as well as the others listed above, is available in both adult and pediatric sizes.

Oxygen-powered breathing device: This device delivers 100% oxygen to a resuscitation mask, an endotracheal tube, an attached mask, or a transtracheal catheter insufflation device. Do not use this mask on children under 12 years of age.

Table 4-3 lists the advantages and disadvantages of oxygen masks.

Suctioning

In the ED, the ET may need to assist in keeping a patient's airway clear of blood, vomit, and other secretions. Suction units consist of the suction source (usually wall suction in the ED), a collection chamber, and thick-walled noncollapsible, wide-bore tubing (see **Figure 4-15**). The tubing must be large enough to allow large particles of matter to pass through and strong enough to prevent kinking, which would result in decreased suction. The tubing must be long enough to easily reach from the suction unit to the patient. A suction catheter fits on the end of the tubing to suction the patient's mouth and/or airway. A common suction catheter is the rigid pharyngeal tip, also called a Yankauer™ or tonsil suction. Long, flexible suction catheters are placed down the patient's airway; therefore, this is considered a **sterile** procedure.

Table 4-3 Summary of Oxygen Therapy Devices

Type of Breathing Device	Oxygen Flow Rate	Oxygen Concentrations	Advantages	Disadvantages
Nasal cannula	2 to 6 L/min	24 to 45%	No rebreathing of expired air	Can be used only on patients who are breathing spontaneously; actual amount of inspired oxygen varies greatly
Face mask	5 to 10 L/min	40 to 60%	Higher oxygen concentration than nasal cannula	Not tolerated well by patients with severe dyspnea; can be used only on patients who are breathing spontaneously
Partial rebreather mask	8 to 12 L/min	50 to 80%	Higher oxygen concentration than nasal cannula or face mask	Must have tight seal on mask; can be used only on patients who are breathing spontaneously; actual amount of inspired oxygen varies greatly
Nonrebreather mask	12 to 15 L/min	85 to 100%	Highest oxygen concentration available by mask	Must have tight seal on mask; do not allow bag to collapse; can be used only on patients who are breathing spontaneously
Venturi mask	2 to 12 L/min	24 to 50%	Oxygen concentration can be adjusted	Can be used only on patients breathing spontaneously
Pocket mask	Exhaled air 10 L/min with adapter	16% 50%	Avoids direct contact with patient's mouth; may add oxygen source; may be used on apneic patient; may be used on children; can obtain excellent tidal volume	Rescuer fatigue
Bag-valve-mask (BVM)	Room air without supplemental oxygen source 12 to 15 L/min	21% 90 to 100%	Quick; oxygen concentration may be increased; rescuer can sense lung compliance; may be used on both apneic and spontaneously breathing patients	Air in stomach; low tidal volume; difficulty obtaining a leak-proof seal
Oxygen-powered breathing device	100 L/min	100%	High oxygen flow, positive pressure; improved lung inflation	Gastric distention; overinflation; standard device cannot be used in children without special adapter; requires an oxygen source

(Reprinted with permission from: McCarthy-Mogan, M. (1999). Advanced life support. In Sheehy, S.B., & Lenehan, G. P. (Eds.). *Manual of emergency care* (5th ed., p. 55). St. Louis, MO: Mosby-Year Book.)

Procedure for Oral Suctioning

- Assemble the equipment and switch on the suction unit.
- Put on gloves and mask.
- Clamp off the suction tubing and make sure the vacuum gauge registers at least 300 mm Hg of pressure then unclamp and continue with the rest of the procedure.
- Attach the tonsil-tip suction.
- Stand by the patient's head.
- Insert the suction tip into the mouth with the convex (bulging) side along the roof of the mouth.
- Insert the tip to the opening of the throat but not into it. Suction for no more than 10 seconds at a time to prevent a decrease in oxygen levels. If secretions plug the tubing section, run water through the tubing until clear.
- The ET does not usually perform suctioning that requires a sterile technique.

Assisting with a Chest Tube Insertion

Patients may require insertion of a chest tube for the removal of air, blood, or fluid from the pleural space in many conditions, including but not limited to:

- <u>Pneumothorax</u>
- <u>Tension pneumothorax</u>
- <u>Hemothorax</u>
- Pleural effusion (a collection of fluid in the pleural space)

When assisting with insertion of a chest tube, it is important to be able to quickly assemble the equipment. The equipment required includes a thoracostomy tray, thoracostomy tube, chest drainage system, suction apparatus, site preparation supplies (sterile saline solution and Betadine™), local anesthetic, suture equipment, 4 × 4 gauze pads, 3 or 4 inch tape, sterile towels, 5- to 10-ml syringes, and sterile gloves (see **Figure 4-16**).

Before insertion, the patient is placed in a sitting position or lying down with the affected side elevated. The patient usually is placed on a cardiac monitor and pulse oximeter as well. Depending on the urgency of the situation, the patient may or may not be sedated before the procedure. The physician almost always administers a local anesthetic to the insertion site. Once the chest tube is inserted and secured by the physician, a dressing with occlusive gauze, 4 × 4 sponges, and 3 or 4 inch tape is applied to secure the insertion site. Never clamp the chest tube.

The usual amount of suction applied to the system is 20 cm H_2O, but 40 to 60 cm H_2O can be used. Some units may have an attached autotransfuser device that allows blood drained from the chest tube to be directly reinfused through an intravenous line into the patient.

After the chest drainage system is set up and working properly, it is important to remember to keep the unit below the level of the chest at all times to prevent complications.

If the patient is to be transported, simply unplug the chest drainage device from the wall suction and allow gravity drainage to occur.

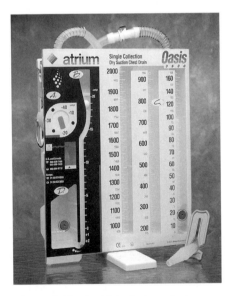

Figure 4-16 Chest Tube Drainage System
(Picture courtesy of Atrium Medical Corporation, Hudson, NH.)

Summary

Respiratory problems should take precedence over any other problems except a blocked or obstructed airway. Intervention and treatment to correct respiratory distress is a priority of the health care team. Understanding the role of the ET in assisting the team in treatment of these patients helps prevent complications and provides a better outcome for the patient.

Bibliography

Emergency Nurses Association. (1998). *Emergency nursing pediatric course Provider Manual* (2nd ed.). Park Ridge, IL: Author.

Seidel, H., Ball, J.W., Dains, J.E., and Benedict, G.W. (1999). *Mosby's guide to physical examination* (4th ed.). St. Louis, MO: Mosby-Year Book.

Sheehy, S., & Lenehan, G. (1999). *Manual of emergency care* (5th ed.). St. Louis, MO: Mosby-Year Book.

Taylor, C., Lyllis, C., & LeMone, P. (1997). *Fundamentals of nursing: The art and science of nursing care* (3rd ed). Philadelphia: Lippincott.

Thomas, C.L. (1997). *Tabor's cyclopedic medical dictionary.* Philadelphia: Davis.

Turner, S.O. (1996). *Competency-based skill building curriculum for unlicensed assistive personnel.* Aliso Viejo, CA: American Association of Critical Care Nurses.

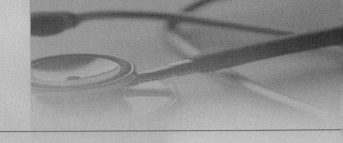

Objectives

Upon completion of this module, the learner should be able to do the following:

- Identify the components of the cardiovascular system.

- Identify life-threatening dysrhythmias of the heart.

- Describe the role of the ET in caring for the patient with a cardiovascular condition.

Chapter 5

Cardiovascular System

Introduction

The circulatory system contains the heart, the arteries, and the veins. The heart is a muscle that pumps blood through the body by contracting and relaxing. Specialized cells in the heart transmit electrical impulses to the heart muscle causing it to contract. Contraction of the heart forces blood out of the heart into the arteries. Arteries carry oxygen-rich blood to tissues while veins carry blood depleted of oxygen back to the heart.

Anatomy and Physiology

The normal adult heart is about the size of a closed fist. It is located slightly to the left of the middle of the chest, between the <u>sternum</u> and the spine. The rib cage protects both the heart and lungs. Below the heart is the diaphragm, the primary muscle of the pulmonary system.

The heart is contained within a fibrous sac called the pericardium. This sac has two layers with a small amount of fluid between each layer. The fluid acts as a lubricant to decrease friction as the heart contracts. These two layers serve to anchor the heart in the chest. Inside the heart are four chambers (see **Figure 5-1**). The <u>atria</u> are the two top chambers, and the <u>ventricles</u> are the two on the bottom. The septum divides the right and left side of the heart. The ventricles are larger and more muscular than the atria. Each ventricle contains two valves. Blood flow through the heart is controlled by the valves, which open to allow blood to flow from one chamber to another and close to prevent blood from flowing back into the heart (see **Figure 5-2**). The top opening of the

Table 5-1 The Electrical Conduction System of the Heart	
Structure	**Function**
Sinoatrial Node (SA Node)	• Located in the left atrium
	• Primary pacemaker cell
	• Sends the signal for the heart to contract
Atrioventricular Node (AV Node)	• Located between the atria and ventricles
	• Passes the electrical impulse along to the ventricles
	• Can also initiate a contraction if the SA node fails
Ventricles	• Electrical impulse then goes to the bundle of His and through Purkinje's fibers to the bottom of the ventricle.

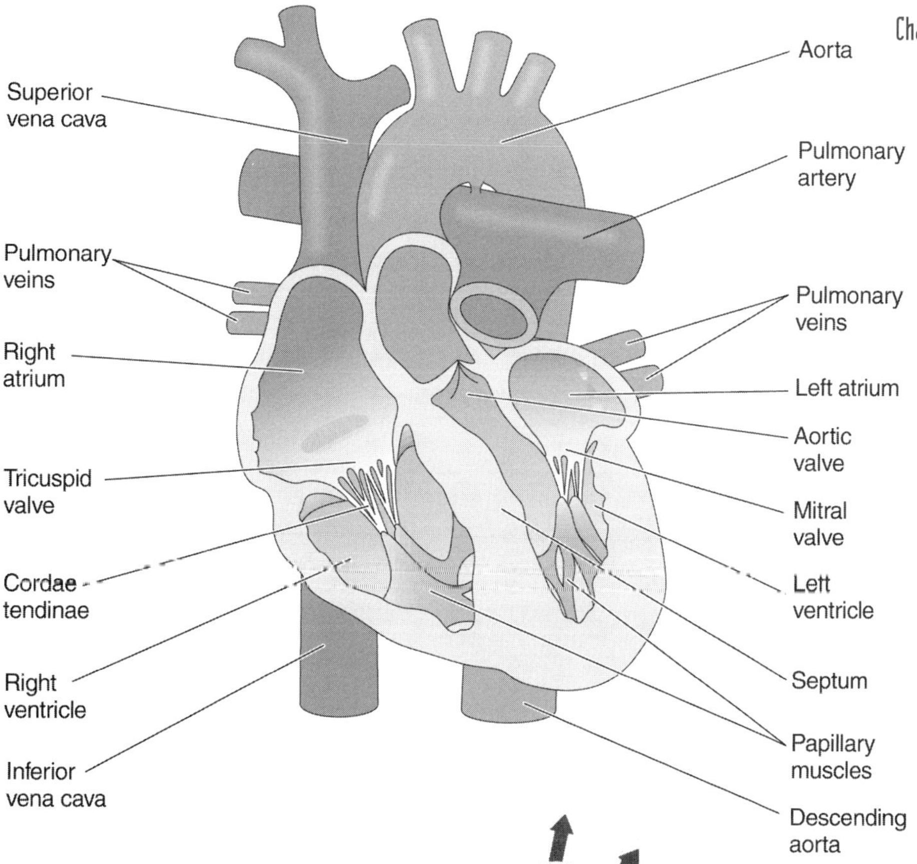

Superior
vena cava

Aorta

Pulmonary
artery

Pulmonary
veins

Right
atrium

Tricuspid
valve

Cordae
tendinae

Right
ventricle

Inferior
vena cava

Pulmonary
veins

Left atrium

Aortic
valve

Mitral
valve

Left
ventricle

Septum

Papillary
muscles

Descending
aorta

Figure 5-1 Anatomy of the Heart

(Reprinted with permission from: Garcia, T.B., and Holtz, N.E. (2001). 12-lead ECG: The art of interpretation. (p. 4) Sudbury.

Aorta

Pulmonary artery

Superior vena cava

Pulmonic valve

Right atrium

Coronary sinus

Tricuspid valve

Inferior vena cava

Right ventricle

Pulmonary veins

Left atrium

Aortic valve

Mitral valve

Left ventricle

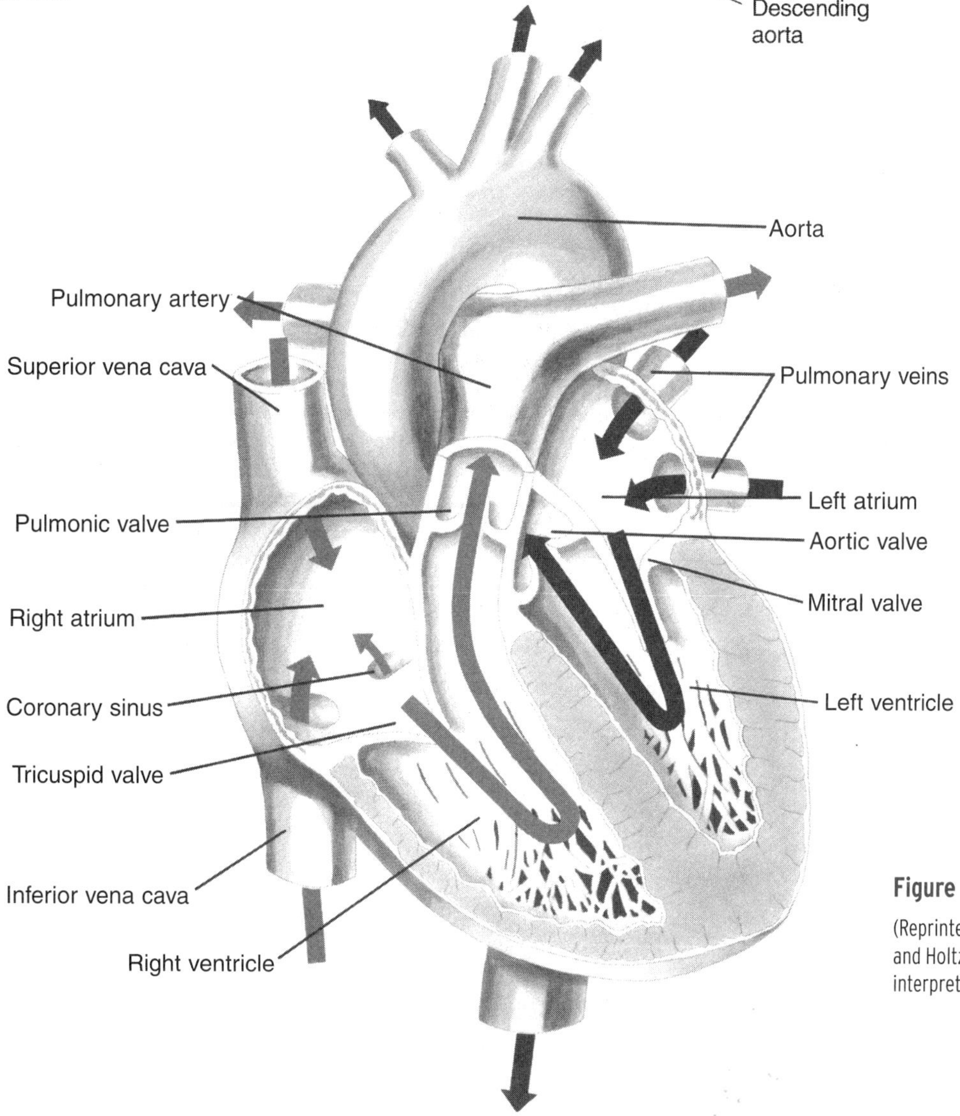

Figure 5-2 Blood Flow Through the Heart

(Reprinted with permission from: Garcia, T.B., and Holtz, N.E. (2001). 12-lead ECG: The art of interpretation. (p. 4) Sudbury.

right atria does not have a valve, so blood flows continuously into the right side of the heart.

Blood circulates through the body and then returns to the heart for oxygenation. The right chambers of the heart receive the deoxygenated blood. The left chambers of the heart contain oxygenated blood received from the lungs. Although atria and ventricles function as one unit, the heart functions as two separate pumps. The right side pumps blood into the pulmonary circulation (the lungs) and the left side pumps blood into the systemic circulation (the body) by way of the aorta.

When the heart muscle contracts, blood pumps through the heart and out into the body and lungs. This action is called <u>systole</u>. After contraction, the heart relaxes. This is called <u>diastole</u>. The atria contract at the same time followed by contraction of the ventricles. The pulse that is felt at the atrial artery (wrist), the carotid artery (neck), or other body sites reflects the pumping action of the heart in the arteries.

Blood Flow to the Heart

Just as body tissues need blood to satisfy their nutritional and oxygenation needs, so do tissues of the heart. The coronary circulation is made up of the arteries and veins that supply blood to the heart muscle. The right and left coronary arteries are the two main arteries. Branches of these arteries supply the entire heart muscle. When the patient has a heart attack (myocardial infarction), one or more of these arteries are blocked and, if not cleared quickly, heart tissue dies. This blockage may interfere with the ability of the heart to pump and may lead to the patient's death.

Normal Cardiac Cycle

The impulse for conduction, generated by the specialized cardiac cells creates small electrical currents (see **Table 5-1, Figure 5-3**). The <u>electrocardiogram</u> (ECG) converts these electrical currents into written form on paper. Different parts of the heart transmit a different looking waveform on the ECG which can be used to identify the effectiveness of the heart and its ability to pump blood through the body.

Selected Cardiac Disorders

Disorders of the cardiac system result from a variety of factors. Some may result from a compromise of the circulatory system, the electrical conduction system, or the pumping action of the heart muscle. Each of these factors is briefly discussed below (see **Table 5-2**).

Circulatory System Compromise

One of the primary causes of a compromised circulatory system is the formation of a clot in an artery and/or vein. A clot results in decreased blood flow through the area. Tissue behind (<u>distal</u> to) the clot does not receive adequate blood flow, oxygen, and nutrients. At this point the tissue begins to die. Signs and symptoms may include pain and difficulty breathing.

Compromise in the Electrical Conduction System

Problems in the electrical conduction system may cause the heart to beat too fast, too slow, or erratically. This type of compromise is detected by the ECG.

Table 5-2 Types of Cardiac Disorders

Disorder	Definition
Coronary Circulation	
Angina	A feeling of pain or a sense of suffocation as a result of an occluded coronary artery
Coronary Artery Disease (CAD)	Fatty deposits that form in the walls of the coronary arteries that eventually grow to a size that occludes the artery
Myocardial Infarction (MI)	An area of tissue in the heart that has died as a result of decreased blood flow and loss of oxygen
Myocardial Ischemia	A local and temporary decrease in blood flow to a tissue area in the heart that may lead to a myocardial infarction
Vascular System	
Peripheral Vascular Disease (PVD)	Changes in the structure of veins and/or arteries resulting in decreased blood flow
Atherosclerosis	Fatty deposits that grow in the walls of vessels that eventually grow to a size that completely occludes the vessel
Embolism	A clot (thrombus) that has broken off from the wall of a vessel and circulates in the blood stream
Thrombosis	Formation of a clot in the wall of a vessel
Electrical Conduction	
Rhythm Disturbances	Alteration in the stimulus of the cells in the cardiac conduction system resulting in an irregular cardiac rhythm (dysrhythmia)
Heart as a Pump	
Cardiac Tamponade	Accumulation of excess fluid in the pericardial sac decreases the ability of the heart to pump
Congestive Heart Failure (CHF)	Inability of the left ventricle to effectively pump blood leads to a backup of fluids systemically
Pericarditis	Inflammation of the pericardium

Pump Compromise

A partially and/or completely occluded (blocked) vessel causes increased pressure in the circulatory system. Increased pressure means the heart must work harder to move the same amount of blood through the system. If the occlusion is not cleared, the heart works even harder and eventually weakens. Chest pain (angina) occurs when there is a lack of oxygen to the heart tissues and may be the first sign of trouble. Chest pain requires immediate attention. The ET may be asked to apply oxygen, obtain blood samples, and perform a 12-lead ECG to assist the health care team in quickly diagnosing the patient and providing the appropriate treatment.

Cardiac Monitoring/Electrocardiogram

The patient's cardiac status may be continuously monitored for rate and rhythm and other abnormalities. Cardiac monitoring may be indicated for chest pain, respiratory distress, chest trauma, or during medication administration. The heart can be monitored in either a three- or five-lead system. A more complete assessment of cardiac electrical activity may be needed, requiring a 12-lead ECG (see **Table 5-3**, **Figure 5-4**). If the patient has a latex allergy, the ET needs to use latex-free electrodes; otherwise, there is no known contraindication to cardiac monitoring or 12-lead ECG.

Tracings recorded during cardiac monitoring represent the electrical activity of the heart. Each complex represents one beat of the heart. By inspecting the complexes individually and collectively, the health care provider assesses cardiac and electrical function. Three distinct waves on the ECG represent the flow of electrical current through the heart as well as contraction of the heart muscle. The P wave represents contraction of the atria, the QRS complex represents contraction of the ventricles, and the T wave represents ventricular recovery (see **Figure 5-7**).

Equipment

- Cardiac monitor/ECG machine with recording paper
- Electrodes
- Alcohol preparation pads

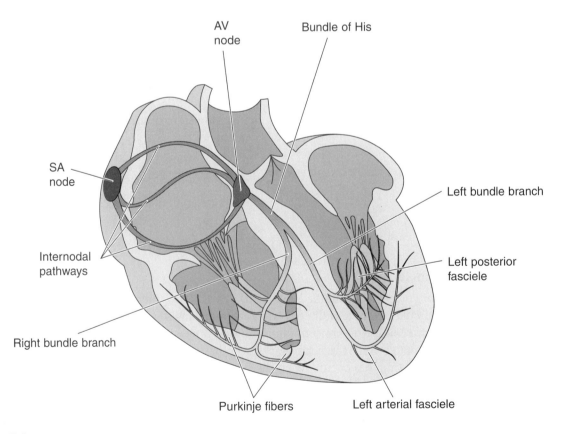

Figure 5-3 Normal Cardiac Cycle

(Reprinted with permission from: Garcia, T.B., and Holtz, N.E. (2001). 12-lead ECG: The art of interpretation. (p. 6) Sudbury.

Table 5-3 Lead II Electrode Placement

Type	Electrode	Placement
Three Electrodes	RA lead (white) or negative lead	• Right anterior chest, below the right clavicle at the midclavicular line
	LA lead (black) or ground lead	• Left anterior chest wall, just below the clavicle at the midclavicular line
	LL lead (red) or positive lead	• Left anterior chest, at lowest palpable rib in the midclavicular line
Five Electrodes	Upper leads	• Same placement for RA and LA leads, as in three-lead placement
	Lower leads Fifth lead (brown)—V_1 in 12-lead ECG	• LL lead in same place, RL (green) on right lower costal margin at anterior axillary line

- Tincture of benzoin so the electrodes can stick to wet or sweaty skin
- Razor to shave off chest hair where the electrodes will go

Considerations when obtaining a 12-lead ECG (see **Figure 5-5**):

- Identify the patient by name and identification bracelet.
- Make the patient comfortable; encourage the patient to relax, to breathe normally, and remain quiet.
- Make sure no other body parts are touching metal or the side rails of the stretcher, because this will distort the tracing.
- Check with the nurse before removing the electrodes, as the patient may require repeat testing.
- Give the ECG tracing to the nurse or physician who ordered it.
- Make sure the patient is in a comfortable position when the recording is completed.
- Document the procedure according to the institution's policy.

Right-sided ECGs or 18-lead ECGs may be indicated for right-sided myocardial infarction or other cardiac problems. The nurse or physician may ask for this type of tracing in addition to the 12-lead type (see **Table 5-4**).

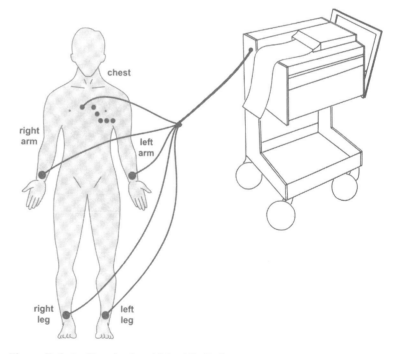

Figure 5-4 Positions for 3- and 5-lead Monitoring

(Reprinted with permission from: Huszar, R. J. (1994). The electrocardiogram. In Huszar, R. J. (Ed.). *Basic dysrhythmias: Interpretation and management* (2nd ed., p. 26). St. Louis, MO: Mosby-Year Book.)

The 12-Lead ECG

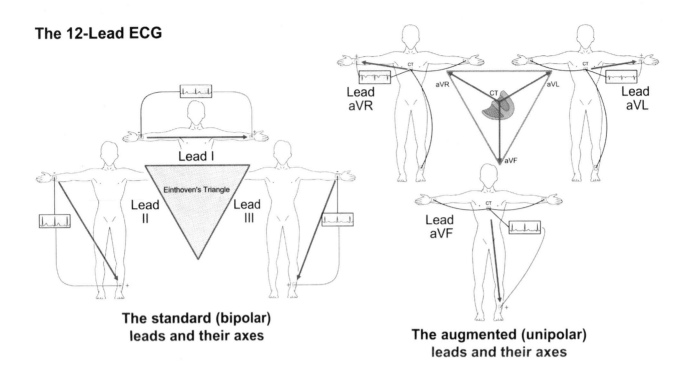

The standard (bipolar) leads and their axes

The augmented (unipolar) leads and their axes

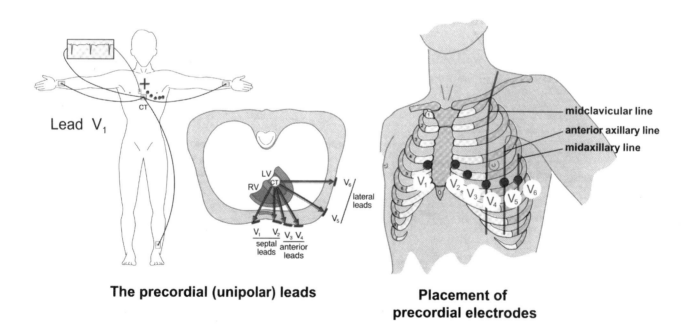

The precordial (unipolar) leads

Placement of precordial electrodes

Figure 5-5A and 5-5B Lead Placement for 12-lead ECG

(Reprinted with permission from: Huszar, R. J. (1995). *Pocket guide to basic dysrhythmias: Interpretation and management.* (Appendix 90-91) St. Louis, MO: Mosby-Year Book.)

Table 5-4 Lead Monitor Positions

Lead	12-Lead ECG Placement	18-Lead or Right-Sided ECG
V_1	Fourth intercostal space, right sternal border	Fourth intercostal space, left sternal border
V_2	Fourth intercostal space, left sternal border	Fourth intercostal space, right sternal border
V_3	Halfway between V_2 and V_4 but not directly below V_2 or directly beside V_4	Halfway between V_2 and V_2. but not directly below V_2 or directly beside V_4.
V_4	Fifth intercostal space, left midclavicular line	Fifth intercostal space, right midclavicular line
V_5	Same level as V_4, left anterior axillary line	Same level as V_4, right anterior axillary line
V_6	Same level as V_4 and V_5, left midaxillary line	Same level as V_4 and V_5, right midaxillary line

Considerations/Troubleshooting

- Place leads in the correct position. Leads that are misplaced can give false readings.
- Avoid placing leads over bony areas.
- If the patient has large breasts, place the electrodes under the breast as close to the heart as possible. The most accurate tracings are obtained through the least amount of fat tissue.
- Apply tincture of benzoin to the electrode sites if the patient is diaphoretic (sweaty). This will help the electrodes adhere to the skin better.
- Shave hair at the electrode site if it interferes with creating good contact between the electrode and skin.
- Sometimes the gel on the back of the electrode dries. If this happens, you will not be able to get a good tracing. Discard old electrodes and use new ones.
- Allow a patient with severe shortness of breath to remain in a position of comfort (sitting upright), and then document this on the patient's ECG record.

Interpretation of Dysrhythmia

A <u>dysrhythmia</u> is a disturbance in the heart rate or rhythm or in the conduction of electrical impulses throughout the heart. Dysrhythmias may be caused by several conditions, such as lack of oxygen (hypoxia), drug intoxication, electrolyte imbalances, and damage to the heart. The disturbance may be single, such as a rapid heart rate, or it may be multiple, such as a rapid rate with conduction delays or premature contractions. The significance of each dysrhythmia depends on the patient's cardiac status and his or her systemic response to the dysrhythmia. Some dysrhythmias are life-threatening, while others cause no great harm to patients throughout their entire life. Interpretation of the ECG is usually performed by the physician or nurse; however, it is important for the ET to be able to identify the life-threatening dysrhythmias, because the ET may be involved in

Figure 5-6 Muscle Tremor ECG and Another Showing Movement

(Reprinted with permission from: Huszar, R. J. (1994). The electrocardiogram. In Huszar, R. J. (Ed.). *Basic dysrhythmias: Interpretation and management* (2nd ed., p. 23). St. Louis, MO: Mosby-Year Book.)

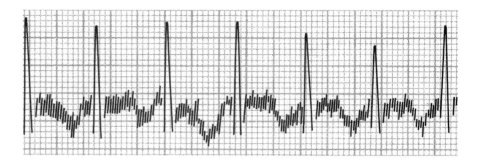

the care of the patient with a cardiac disorder. If an abnormality is identified, report this immediately to the nurse or physician for further evaluation and treatment.

Before identifying the abnormalities, it is important to be able to recognize what a normal heartbeat looks like on the ECG tracing and to know the normal ranges of the patient's vital signs. Once the norms are known, it is easier to recognize when something does not look "quite right." This quick response usually results in early intervention and appropriate treatment for the patient.

After placing the monitor leads on the patient, turn on the monitor and look at the waveform. Traditionally, the patient is monitored in Lead II, although the ET will need to check with the individual institutional policy. Some waves may look abnormal but are caused by improper placement or patient movement (see **Figure 5-6**).

Normal Sinus Rhythm (NSR) is seen upright when viewed in Leads II and V_1 on the cardiac monitor (see **Figure 5-7**). A normal heart rate for an adult is 60 to 100/bpm. Check to make sure the patient's palpated pulse corresponds to the heart rate the monitor is showing. If the two are different, check the leads to make sure they are attached correctly, and then notify the nurse with these findings. In normal sinus rhythm, the rhythm is regular and the distance between each beat is the same. There is a P wave that precedes QRS complex with each beat. The P waves should be small and rounded; the QRS complex should be pointing up (in Lead II and V_1) and be fairly narrow. The T wave should follow the QRS complex and also be pointing upright and larger than the P wave.

If the patient's waveform does not follow the characteristics of a normal sinus rhythm, the nurse should be notified immediately. Potentially life-threatening dysrhythmias to identify are Premature Ventricular Contractions (PVCs), Ventricular Tachycardia (V-Tach or VT), Ventricular Fibrillation (V-Fib or VF), and Asystole.

Premature Ventricular Contractions

Premature ventricular contractions (PVC) may occur in seemingly healthy persons; however, they are more common when the heart is diseased or injured. With this dysrhythmia, the ventricles are stimulated prematurely (early) and contract prematurely. PVCs rarely occur in a child or infant. On the ECG, a PVC appears as a wide, bizarre-shaped QRS complex with no preceding P wave (see **Figure 5-8**). Often the QRS complex points in the opposite direction from the patient's normal QRS complexes. The T wave that follows is also wider and larger, and usually points in the opposite direction from the QRS complex. The more frequently PVCs occur, the greater the risk of developing a life-threatening rhythm.

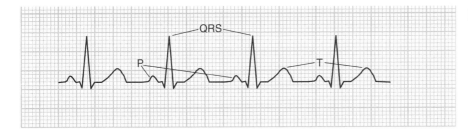

Rate:	60–100 BPM
Regularity:	Regular
P wave:	Present
P:QRS ratio:	1:1
PR interval:	Normal
QRS width:	Normal
Grouping:	None
Dropped beats:	None

Putting it all together:
This rhythm represents the normal state with the SA node as the lead pacer. The intervals should all be consistent and within the normal range. Note that this refers to the atrial rate; normal sinus rhythm (NSR) can occur with a ventricular escape rhythm or other ventricular abnormality if AV dissociation exists.

Figure 5-7 Normal Sinus Rhythm

(Reprinted with permission from: Garcia, T.B., and Holtz, N.E., (2001). *12-lead ECG: The art of interpretation.* (p. 55) Sudbury.

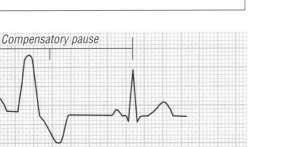

Rate:	Depends on the underlying rhythm
Regularity:	Irregular
P wave:	Not present on the PVC
P:QRS ratio:	No P waves on the PVC
PR interval:	None
QRS width:	Wide (>0.12 seconds), bizarre appearance
Grouping:	Usually not present
Dropped beats:	None

Putting it all together:
A PVC is caused by the premature firing of a ventricular cell. The ventricular pacer fires before the normal SA node or supraventricular pacer, which causes the ventricles to be in a refractory state (not yet repolarized and unavailable to fire again) when the normal pacer fires. Hence, the ventricles do not contract at their normal time. However, the underlying pacing schedule is not altered, so the beat following the PVC will arrive on time. This is called a *compensatory pause.*

Figure 5-8 Strip of PVC

(Reprinted with permission from: Garcia, T.B., and Holtz, N.E., (2001). *12-lead ECG: The art of interpretation.* (p. 63) Sudbury.

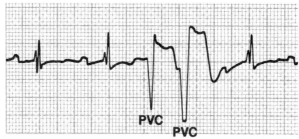

paired PVCs (multifocal PVCs)

Figure 5-9 ECG Tracing Showing Couplets

(Reprinted with permission from: Huszar, R. J. (1994). Ventricular arrhythmias. In Huszar, R. J. (Ed.). *Basic dysrhythmias: Interpretation and management* (2nd ed., p. 169). St. Louis, MO: Mosby-Year Book.)

When two PVCs occur right next to each other, they are called "couplets" (see **Figure 5-9**).

When a PVC occurs after every normal-looking beat, it is known as bigeminy. Trigeminy occurs when a PVC occurs after every second normal-looking beat (see **Figure 5-10**).

When two or more PVCs occur in a row and are followed by resumption of a normal-looking rhythm, it is referred to as a burst, run of, or salvos of ventricular tachycardia (see **Figure 5-11**).

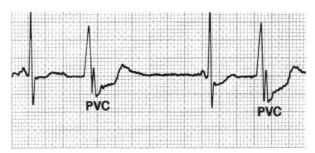

bigeminy (unifocal PVCs)

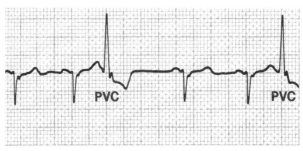

trigeminy (unifocal PVCs)

Figure 5-10 ECG Tracing Showing Bigeminy and Trigeminy

(Reprinted with permission from: Huszar, R. J. (1994). Ventricular arrhythmias. In Huszar, R. J. (Ed.). *Basic dysrhythmias: Interpretation and management* (2nd ed., p. 169). St. Louis, MO: Mosby-Year Book.)

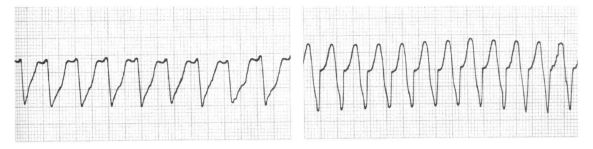

Figure 5-11 Run of V-Tach

(Reprinted with permission from: Huszar, R. J. (1994). Ventricular arrhythmias. In Huszar, R. J. (Ed.). *Basic dysrhythmias: Interpretation and management* (2nd ed., p. 173). St. Louis, MO: Mosby-Year Book.)

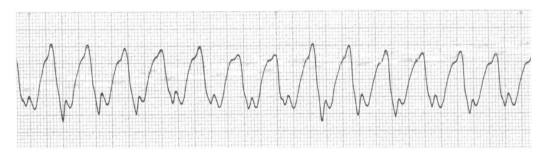

Figure 5-12 A strip of Ventricular Tachycardia

(Reprinted with permission from: Huszar, R. J. (1994). Ventricular arrhythmias. In Huszar, R. J. (Ed.). *Basic dysrhythmias: Interpretation and management* (2nd ed., p. 173). St. Louis, MO: Mosby-Year Book.)

Ventricular Tachycardia (V-tach)

In many cases PVCs precipitate ventricular tachycardia. This dysrhythmia can be identified by wide, but uniform, QRS complexes and a regular rhythm (see **Figure 5-12**). A patient may or may not have a palpable pulse with V-tach. The patient without a pulse is treated with immediate defibrillation by the physician or nurse. Patients in V-tach who still have a pulse are not able to tolerate high ventricular rates for long; they must be treated immediately with drugs, **defibrillation**, or a combination of both.

Ventricular Fibrillation

Ventricular fibrillation (VF or V-fib) appears as an uncoordinated tracing without any type of pattern (see **Figure 5-13**). The patient has no palpable pulse and appears dead. The heart is not contracting but is quivering, which some describe as looking like a "bag of worms." The only effective treatment for this condition is immediate defibrillation.

Asystole

Asystole is also known as ventricular standstill or cardiac arrest. The ability to survive this condition, as with all life-threatening conditions, depends not only on the medical care given, but also on the condition of the patient's heart muscle, and the function of the pulmonary system.

Asystole means "absence of contraction." The heart does not beat and does not move at all. It typically appears on the monitor as a fairly straight line (see **Figure 5-14**). Before deciding that the tracing truly shows asystole,

Ventricular Fibrillation (VF)

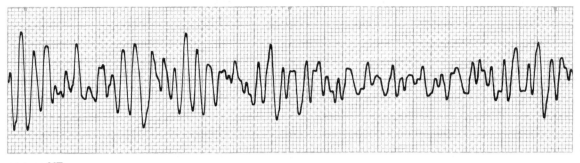

coarse VF

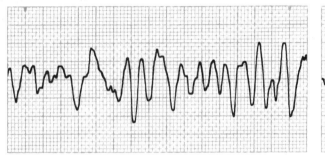

coarse VF

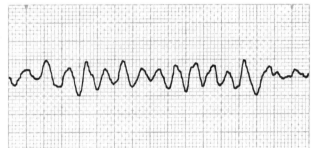

coarse VF

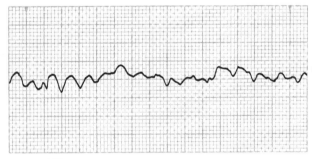

coarse VF

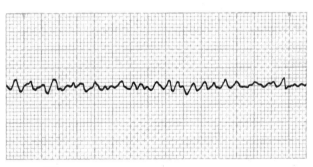

coarse VF

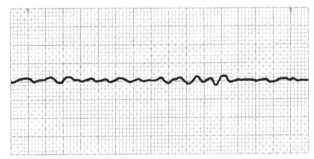

fine VF

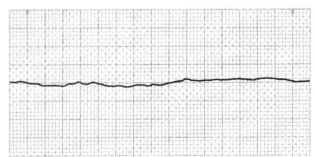

fine VF

Figure 5-13 Ventricular Fibrillation

(Reprinted with permission from: Huszar, R. J. (1994). Ventricular arrhythmias. In Huszar, R. J. (Ed.). *Basic dysrhythmias: Interpretation and management* (2nd ed., p. 179). St. Louis, MO: Mosby-Year Book.)

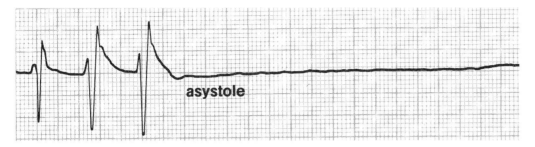

Figure 5-14 Asystole

(Reprinted with permission from: Huszar, R. J. (1994). Ventricular arrhythmias. In Huszar, R. J. (Ed.). *Basic dysrhythmias: Interpretation and management* (2nd ed., p. 185). St. Louis, MO: Mosby-Year Book.)

remember to check the patient, the leads, and the rhythm in another lead on the cardiac monitor before calling for the resuscitation team.

Treatment of asystole begins with cardiopulmonary resuscitation (CPR). The physician attempts to determine the cause for the asystole and treats the underlying cause. The ET may be involved in assisting with placement of an external **pacemaker** or performing chest compressions.

External Pacemaker

When a patient requires an external pacemaker to maintain the rate of cardiac contractions, the ET may be requested to apply the external pacer pads. One pad is placed on the **anterior** chest wall, and the second is placed on the patient's back according to the specific manufacturer's instructions. Place the pads so that the current passes straight through the chest cavity. Many external pacer pads have multiple functions and also can be used for defibrillation, **cardioversion**, and cardiac monitoring.

Summary

The role of the ET in caring for a patient with a cardiovascular disorder may vary widely. The ET must be able to identify the norms of the cardiovascular system so that when an abnormality occurs it is quickly reported so immediate action may be taken. Once heart muscle dies, as in a myocardial infarction, it cannot be regenerated, and the heart suffers permanent damage. The ET participates in many of the diagnostic studies related to cardiovascular problems and should be able to recognize life-threatening situations.

Bibliography

Seidel, H., Ball, J.W., Dains, J.E., and Benedict, G.W. (1999). *Mosby's guide to physical examination* (4th ed.). St. Louis, MO: Mosby-Year Book.

Sheehy, S., & Lenehan, G. (1999). *Manual of emergency care* (5th ed.). St. Louis, MO: Mosby-Year Book.

Taylor, C., Lyllis, C., & LeMone, P. (1997). *Fundamentals of nursing: The art and science of nursing care* (3rd ed.). Philadelphia: Lippincott.

Thomas, C.L. (1997). *Tabor's cyclopedic medical dictionary.* Philadelphia: Davis.

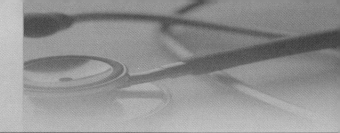

Chapter 6

Upon completion of this module, the learner should be able to do the following:

- Define populations at risk for trauma.

- Identify the Emergency Technician's (ET) role and responsibilities in the care of the trauma patient.

- List equipment needed for patient transfers.

Trauma

Introduction

In the emergency department (ED), the ET is involved with patients who are the victims of trauma. Trauma may be defined as an injury to the human body, either intentional or unintentional, occurring through the body's interaction with the environment. Emergency trauma patients may have a single injury, such as a lacerated finger, or injuries involving multiple body systems.

It is estimated that nearly 60 million injuries occur annually in the United States. A thorough knowledge of the role and types of skills needed helps the ET to safely assist in the care of the trauma patient.

Mechanisms of a Traumatic Injury

Mechanism of injury refers to the conditions under which a person is injured. The severity of the mechanism of injury may be related to the type of agent used to cause the injury, as well as the environmental conditions and the patient's physical and mental status. The area/location where a person lives may increase his or her risk for certain types of trauma. For example, a person who lives in an agricultural region has a higher chance of sustaining trauma from farm machinery than someone who lives in an urban area.

Examples of mechanisms of injury include the following:
- Motor vehicle crashes.
- Falls.
- Penetrating injury: Sharp instruments and firearms.
- Blunt injury.
- Exposure to heat or burn injury.
- Drowning.
- Electrical injury.
- Radiation.

Patient Population

Trauma is the leading cause of death in persons under 44 years of age. Motor vehicle crashes (MVCs) are the leading cause of death in persons 1 to 34 years of age. In the pediatric population, trauma is responsible for more than half of all deaths.

Risk factors associated with trauma include the following:
- Age.
- Gender: Males are at higher risk.

- Income: In a depressed economy, the suicide and homicide rates rise while motor vehicle crashes decrease.

- Alcohol use: Associated with 63% of all motor vehicle crashes in persons 21 to 34 years of age.

- Geography: Urban versus rural concerns in types of injury. Homicides and suicides are highest in urban areas.

- Temporal concerns (time): Trauma deaths occur most frequently on weekends. Unintentional injuries are most common in July with summer-related activities.

Trauma Resuscitation

The goal in trauma resuscitation is to quickly assess and identify all life-threatening injuries. Once identified, these conditions must be treated and the patient stabilized. While the ET is not responsible for patient assessment, a general knowledge of the resuscitation routine helps the ET to successfully participate as a member of the team. The trauma response is a standardized, systematic approach that ensures that no injuries are missed. The two major components of standardized trauma care are the primary and secondary assessments. The primary assessment involves evaluating Airway, Breathing, Circulation, and Disability (neurologic status)—A-B-C-D—of the patient while maintaining cervical spine stabilization and/or immobilization (also called spinal precautions). The goal of the primary assessment is to identify and treat all life-threatening injuries.

The secondary assessment is a continuation of the systematic approach in an effort to identify all areas of injuries. The secondary assessment consists of the following:

E = Expose/Environmental control

F = Full set of vital signs/Five interventions/Family presence

G = Give comfort measures

H = Head-to-toe assessment/History

I = Inspect posterior surfaces

The mnemonic, A-B-C-D-E-F-G-H-I, is used as a way to remember all components of the primary and secondary assessments. In the hospital setting, the primary and secondary assessments are performed by the physician or nurse.

The Primary Assessment

A is for Airway, with simultaneous cervical spine stabilization and/or immobilization

The airway is assessed to ensure it is open, or patent. Think of the airway as the tube that runs from the mouth to the lungs. This must be clear for the patient to breathe. The trauma patient may require the jaw thrust or chin lift maneuver to open the airway, as opposed to **hyperextending** the neck because of the risk of cervical spine injury (see **Figure 6-1** and **Figure 6-2**). Never use the head tilt maneuver to open the airway in a trauma patient as it may cause further damage to the cervical spine.

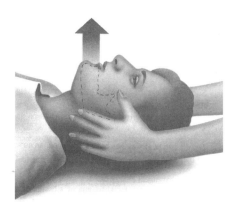

Figure 6-1 Jaw Thrust Maneuver

(Reprinted with permission from: Emergency Nurses Association. (2000). Airway and ventilation Interventions skill station. In *Trauma nursing core course provider manual* (5th ed., p. 364). Des Plaines, IL: Author.)

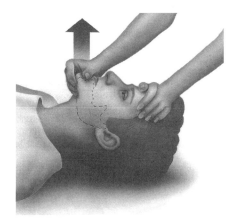

Figure 6-2 Chin Lift Maneuver

(Reprinted with permission from: Emergency Nurses Association. (2000). Airway and ventilation Interventions skill station. In *Trauma nursing core course provider manual* (5th ed., p. 364). Des Plaines, IL: Author.)

Figure 6-3 Spinal Immobilization

(Reproduced with permission from: French, J.P. (1995). Stabilization procedures. In French, J.P. (Ed.). *Pediatric emergency skills.* (p. 141) St. Louis, MO: Mosby-Year Book)

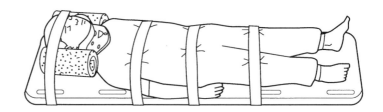

Suctioning the mouth also may be required to clear the airway of existing blood or vomit. **<u>Spinal precautions</u>** must be maintained in all trauma patients until injury to the spinal cord is ruled out. This includes patients with mechanisms of injury such as falls, motor vehicle crashes, and penetrating injuries to the upper body, head, or areas in which the path of the penetrating object could have injured the spinal cord. Spinal stabilization includes the use of long backboards, rigid cervical collars, and side immobilization devices for the head (see **Figure 6-3**). The goal of therapy is to prevent further injury to the spinal cord by preventing motion. The ET may assist with the application of these devices.

B is for Breathing

Assess breathing by looking for the rise and fall of the patient's chest and the rate and effort of breathing. Check to see if the patient is making unusual noises while breathing or if breathing is irregular. Report any breathing problems to the nurse immediately. Look at color of the skin and check if the lips, ear tips, nose is cyanotic (blue). This is also a sign of not enough oxygen in the bloodstream and supplemental oxygen is needed. Notify the physician or nurse if the color of the patient looks at all abnormal. A bag-valve-mask (BVM) device may be used to help deliver oxygen to the trauma patient. Apply supplemental oxygen to all trauma patients under direction of the nurse or physician. Refer to Chapter 4: Respiratory System for a discussion on oxygen therapy devices.

C is for Circulation

The circulation is quickly determined by feeling for the presence of a pulse either in the neck (carotid), wrist (radial), or groin (femoral). Also assess the patient's level of consciousness (awareness), skin color, and temperature. In addition, the trauma team also notes any excessive bleeding from wounds and takes appropriate action.

D is for Disability (Neurologic Status)

The physician or nurse notes the patient's response to pain and state of alertness. The pupils of the eyes are checked for size and response to light. The patient's ability to move his or her arms and legs and to feel touch is also determined. Any abnormality may indicate injury to the brain or spinal cord.

The Secondary Assessment

E is for Expose/Environmental control (Remove clothing and keep patient warm)

It is important to undress (or expose) the patient to look for any additional injuries. Typically, very sharp scissors are used to cut off the clothing, thereby reducing the risk of moving the patient who may have a spinal cord injury.

Once undressed, the patient can rapidly become cold or hypothermic, which may cause additional complications. Apply warm blankets and provide privacy. Maintain a trauma room temperature of at least 26.7°C (80°F). The pediatric and geriatric population are extremely sensitive to cold, and extra care must be taken to prevent heat loss in the ED. In this case, overhead heating lamps may be used.

F is for Full set of vital signs/Five interventions/Family presence

The ET may be responsible for obtaining vital signs. The initial set of vital signs serves as a baseline measurement. In the severely injured patient, blood pressure, pulse, and respirations are obtained at 5-minute intervals for the first 20 to 30 minutes or until the patient is stabilized; then, every 15 to 30 minutes thereafter or as directed by the nurse.

Core body temperature must be obtained as well. If the patient has an abnormal body temperature, expect to continue monitoring this vital sign frequently. Avoid the use of rectal temperature measurements in those patients with head injuries.

Record vital signs and verbally report them to the physician and nurse caring for the patient. Avoid taking blood pressure readings in an injured arm or one with an IV, if possible, as these may impede flow of the solution. Count pulses and heart rate for a full minute.

Additional interventions include placing cardiac monitor leads and pulse oximetry on the patient. Lead II usually is used to monitor the heart. To place leads for Lead II monitoring, use the mnemonics "white on right" and "smoke over fire" to help remember that the white electrode is placed on the patient's right upper chest; the black electrode is placed on the left upper chest; and the red electrode is placed on the lower left side of the trunk. Additional information on cardiac monitoring is included in chapter 5: Cardiovascular System.

The pulse oximeter is an indirect way of measuring how well the patient is being oxygenated (oxygen saturation). The probe is usually placed on the finger of an adult. Some types of pulse oximeter probes may be placed on the earlobe, nose, or toes of children. Additional information on pulse oximetry is included in chapter 3: Vital Signs.

An indwelling urinary catheter and gastric tube may or may not be inserted at this time based on the patient's condition. These would be placed under direction of the nurse or physician.

The F is also for family presence. A health care professional is assigned to provide explanations about procedures and to be with the family while they are in the ED.

G is for Give Comfort Measures

Comfort measures include pain management (pharmacologic analgesia), alternative pain control (touch, positioning, relaxation techniques), verbal reassurance, listening to the patient, and establishing a trusting relationship with the patient.

H is for History and Head-to-Toe Assessment

A history is obtained from the patient, family members, or prehospital personnel who brought the patient to the ED. The mechanism of injury, and any past medical history are important factors in trauma patient care. A head-to-toe assessment is done to identify all other injuries.

I is for Inspect Posterior Surfaces

Trauma patients most often arrive in the ED secured to a backboard. It is important that the assessment of the patient also includes checking the back for additional areas of injury. The ET may assist with turning the patient.

Role of the Emergency Technician

The role of the ET in trauma care is that of an assistant to the RN on the trauma team. Depending on your state (for scope of practice issues) and the policies established by the hospital, the ET may be expected to:

- Prepare the trauma room for arrival of the patient, gather needed equipment, clean and restock room after the trauma resuscitation has occurred.

- Perform CPR, as needed.

- Measure and record vital signs.

- Place leads for cardiac monitoring.

- Place pulse oximetry probe.

- Assist with spinal stabilization.

- Collect laboratory specimens.

- Insert urinary catheter (refer to the scope of practice in the state).

- Undress or expose the patient.

- Provide wound care.

- Assist with splinting.

- Assist transport of patient to x-ray, operating room, or admission.

- Perform runner activities, including getting supplies or equipment.

Trauma Room Set-Up

Advance preparation is key in the care of the trauma patient. Accessibility of equipment and readiness saves valuable seconds in the resuscitation of a severely injured trauma victim. In the case of upper airway obstruction, having the necessary equipment ready and available makes the difference in the patient's ultimate survival. Careful and thorough preparation of the trauma room is invaluable. Restocking the room after each trauma provides the life-saving equipment that every trauma patient may need (see **Figure 6-4**).

Some of the specific equipment and conditions that must be in place before the arrival of the patient include the following:

- Adequate barrier protection apparel including: gowns, gloves, goggles, masks, booties, and caps for the trauma team

- Lead shields, including lead aprons and thyroid shields for both the patient and the staff

- Adjust the room temperature to 26.7°C (80°F) to help prevent hypothermia in the trauma patient.

- Make sure the wall suction unit works and tonsil-tip and tracheal suction catheters are available.

- Be sure wall oxygen is set up and there is a full portable oxygen tank under the stretcher.

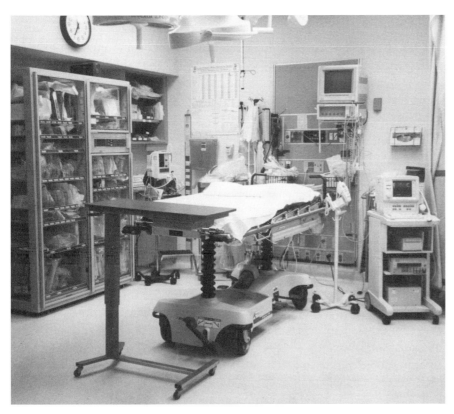

Figure 6-4 Trauma Room

(Provided courtesy of Donna Massey, RN, MSN, CCNS.)

- Available airway equipment including a bag-valve-mask device, oropharyngeal and nasopharyngeal airways, intubation equipment with endotracheal tubes of various sizes and a 10-ml syringe

- A portable monitor or defibrillator, electrocardiogram electrodes, defibrillator pads (if used in the facility), or gel for defibrillation. Also make sure there is plenty of paper in the defibrillator to record electrical activity. Ensure that the batteries in the defibrillator are fully charged and that there are batteries available as a backup. This piece of equipment should be plugged into an electrical outlet at all times as conditions permit.

- Pulse oximetry and appropriate size probe

- Doppler, blood pressure cuff, rectal thermometer

- Paper or forms for recording the trauma resuscitation (hospital-specific)

- Adequate supply of warm blankets and warm IV fluid bags

- Other supplies as requested by the nurse (i.e., fluid warmer, ventilator, body warming or cooling devices, splints, chest tube)

- Garbage cans/receptacles for trash

- Patient valuables/garment bag for items removed from the patient and secured

- Stands or trays to bring near the bedside for supplies (i.e., Mayo™ stands)

Additional Duties

The ET also may be expected to obtain blood samples from the trauma patient. These patients frequently arrive with IVs in their arms, so blood draws must be done below the IV site, not above it. Drawing blood at or above the IV site dilutes the blood specimen with extra IV solution going in. Try to access the vein at least 6 inches below the IV site to prevent possible dilution of the sample. The blood collection tube used for "type and crossmatch" must be given priority in the event that a blood transfusion is necessary. A blood alcohol content level (BAC) may be drawn to differentiate someone who is intoxicated from someone with a head injury. Use povidine iodine wipes to clean the skin instead of alcohol when drawing a BAC so the results are not contaminated.

If the ET is allowed to catheterize the trauma patient (per facility protocol), there are several special considerations. Never insert a catheter into a patient who has blood at the urinary meatus (opening). In the male trauma patient, a urinary catheter must not be placed until after a rectal examination has been done by the physician. This allows the physician to assess for possible injury to the urethra by his or her ability to feel the prostate gland. Placing a catheter into a damaged urethra may cause serious complications for the patient. Trauma patients with obvious injury to the external genitalia must not have a urinary catheter placed.

The general principles of wound care apply to the trauma patient. The goal of therapy is to prevent further tissue damage and infection. Wounds are cleansed, according to institutional protocol. Bleeding may be controlled through use of direct pressure by placing a gloved hand over a dressing, raising the extremity above the level of the heart, or using **pressure points**.

Assisting with Splinting of Extremities

Limit handling of a fractured (broken) extremity to prevent further injury. Movement of a fractured extremity also causes the patient pain. Immobilization serves to decrease bleeding, nerve injury, and pain. If the ET is asked to move a fractured extremity, support it above and below the fracture. Immobilize the joint above and below the fracture site, as well, to protect the injured area. Cover all open wounds around the fracture site with a sterile dressing because an open wound is an entry site for microorganisms that may cause infection to the bone. Do not push exposed or protruding bone ends back into the open wound as this may cause further injury to the bone, nerves, or blood vessels surrounding the fracture.

Always check the pulse below the fracture site, and note skin temperature and movement before *and* after splinting. Elevate splinted extremities on a pillow and apply ice to decrease swelling. See Chapter 9: Musculoskeletal Emergencies for further information.

Patient Transfer Assistance

The trauma patient may require tests to identify internal injuries that cannot be done in the trauma room. Computerized tomography (CT) scans, magnetic resonance imaging (MRI), or other specialized tests may be needed. Moving an unstable patient from one location to another requires careful planning and preparation. The same life-support equipment required in the ED also may be needed in an elevator or hallway when moving the patient. While away from the ED for these types of additional tests, the following equipment should be transported with the patient (at a minimum):

- Blood pressure cuff (manual)
- Pulse oximetry (portable)
- Cardiac monitor or defibrillator and a supply of batteries
- Portable suction and supply of catheters
- Extra IV solution bags
- Extra dressings, tape, and clean gloves
- Oxygen tank and airway devices
- Portable IV poles or IV pumps
- Other supplies/equipment as indicated by the nurse or physician

Transferring a trauma patient is a team effort. Moving a trauma patient from a stretcher to an x-ray table must be done while keeping the spine immobilized, if injury to the spine has not yet been ruled out. The trauma patient with critical injuries has many IV lines and tubes; therefore, it is important to ensure that the lines are secured so that they are not accidentally pulled out.

Summary

Successful resuscitation of the trauma patient requires a teamwork approach. As a valued member of the trauma team, the ET is expected to perform specific tasks and assist other members of the team in caring for the trauma patient to ensure that further injury does not occur, with the best possible outcome for the trauma patient.

Bibliography

Collier, I. C., Heitkemper, M., & Lewis, S. M. (1996). *Medical surgical nursing: Assessment and management of clinical problems* (4th ed.). St. Louis, MO: Mosby-Year Book.

Emergency Nurses Association. (2000). *Trauma nursing core course (provider manual)* (5th ed.). Des Plaines, IL: Author.

Kidd, P., & Stuart, P. (1996). *Mosby's emergency nursing reference.* St. Louis, MO: Mosby-Year Book.

McQuillan, K.A., Von Rueden, K.T., Hartsock, R.L., Flynn, M.B., and Whalen, E. (2002). *Trauma nursing from resuscitation through rehabilitation* (3rd ed.). Philadelphia: Saunders.

Porter, W. (1996). *Porter's pocket guide to critical care* (5th ed.). Chicago: Porter and Associates.

Upon completion of this module, the learner should be able to do the following:

- Describe the role of the ET in caring for the patient with head and neck emergencies.

- List three common tests and procedures performed in the ED related to head and neck injuries.

- State the essential elements of a neurologic observation.

Chapter 7

Head and Neck Emergencies

Introduction

Head injuries are the leading cause of death in the United States. Head injuries may result from falls, gunshot wounds, stabbings, and motor vehicle crashes. Stroke or "brain attack" is the third leading cause of death.

Head and neck emergencies are extremely frightening for both the patient and the family. The real or perceived loss of the ability to move one's arms or legs, communicate, and be a contributing member of society makes caring for this type of patient a challenge for the health care team.

Anatomy of the Nervous System

The three components of the nervous system are the central nervous system (CNS), the peripheral nervous system (PNS), and the autonomic nervous system (ANS). Each plays a vital role in bodily functions. The CNS includes the brain and spinal cord and is covered and protected by the bones of the skull and vertebrae. The PNS includes all of the nerves and ganglia outside the brain and spinal cord. Finally, the ANS controls all involuntary functions, such as the glands, cardiac and smooth muscle, respiratory system, and the skin.

The Brain

The brain can be divided into three different areas: the cerebrum, cerebellum, and brain stem (see **Figure 7-1**). The cerebrum, the largest area of the brain, is composed of two cerebral hemispheres that are divided into frontal, parietal, temporal, and occipital lobes. Each lobe performs specific functions, which are described in **Table 7-1**.

The cerebellum, another section of the brain, is much smaller than the cerebrum. The cerebellum is responsible for body movement and coordination.

The brain stem is the structure the brain sits on. It acts as the relay station or pathway for messages to travel between the brain and the spinal cord. The most important nerve centers for consciousness, respiratory, and cardiac functions are located in the brain stem.

Head Injuries

Head injuries occur from either blunt or penetrating trauma. Blunt injuries, such as from a blow to the head, falls, or motor vehicle crashes (MVCs), may result in skull fractures and damage to the brain tissue. Concussions, contusions, and venous and arterial bleeding also are possible injuries that may result from blunt trauma to the head. Penetrating injuries such as gunshot wounds may result in the same type of brain damage. Patients with minor head injuries may be discharged from the ED after a thorough exam-

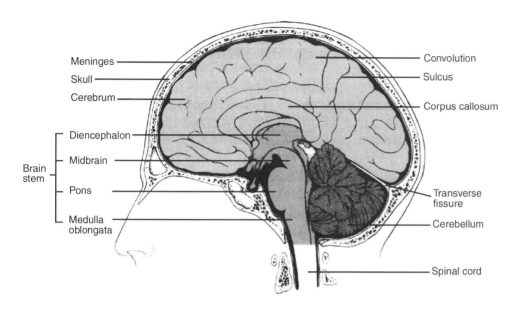

Meninges
Skull
Cerebrum

Diencephalon
Brain stem
Midbrain
Pons
Medulla oblongata

Convolution
Sulcus
Corpus callosum

Transverse fissure
Cerebellum

Spinal cord

Figure 7-1 Brain Structures.

(Reprinted with permission from: Hole, J.W. (1993). *Human anatomy and physiology* (6th ed.). Dubuque, IA: Wm. C. Brown. Reprinted with permission of Times Mirror Higher Education Group, Inc., Dubuque, IA. All Rights Reserved.)

ination and observation for potential complications. Minor lacerations to the scalp may require suturing or stapling by the physician (see chapter 10, Surface Trauma). Severe head injuries require hospital admission and possibly surgery. Patients with head injuries need close monitoring using the Glasgow Coma Scale (GCS) or other neurologic assessment tools for tracking and trending changes in condition.

Impaled objects to the head should be stabilized (never remove an impaled object) and the patient taken to surgery so that the object can be removed in a controlled setting.

Patients who sustain a head injury should be treated as though they have associated injuries to the neck and spine.

Table 7-1 Function and Location of the Lobes

Lobes of the Cerebrum	Location	Function
Frontal lobe	Anterior portion of the cerebral cortex	• Higher intellectual abilities • Voluntary muscle control • Formation of words and speech
Parietal lobe	Upper central lobe of the cerebral cortex	• Awareness of position and touch, sensitivity to heat, cold, pain • Integration and coordination of sensory information
Occipital lobe	Posterior portion of the cerebrum	• Vision
Temporal lobe	Lower side portion of the cerebrum	• Hearing, taste, and smell • Interprets sounds as words • Memory center

The Spinal Cord

The spinal cord is actually a continuation of the brain and is approximately 17 inches in length. There is an opening at the base of the skull called the foramen magnum through which the spinal cord exits. This major portion of the CNS transmits information to and from the brain.

The spinal cord is protected by the vertebral column, or spine (see **Figure 7-2**). The spine consists of 33 bones called vertebra. The spine is organized into five sections, listed here is order from the neck to the tailbone: Cervical, thoracic, lumbar, sacral, and coccyx. Ligaments hold the vertebra together and limit motion of the vertebra. Cartilaginous discs between the vertebra act as shock absorbers for the spine (see **Figure 7-3**).

Spinal Cord Injuries

Injury can occur to the vertebral column alone or in conjunction with injury to the spinal cord. Injury to the spinal cord may result in partial, temporary, or permanent loss of bodily functions of both voluntary and involuntary muscles.

Mechanisms of injury include blunt or penetrating trauma, or a combination of both. Examples include falls (such as landing on the feet after falling off a roof), MVCs, stabbings, gunshot wounds, and sports injuries. There is also the potential to "extend" the degree of injury if the ET and other members of the health care team do not maintain spinal cord immobilization during transfers and examinations.

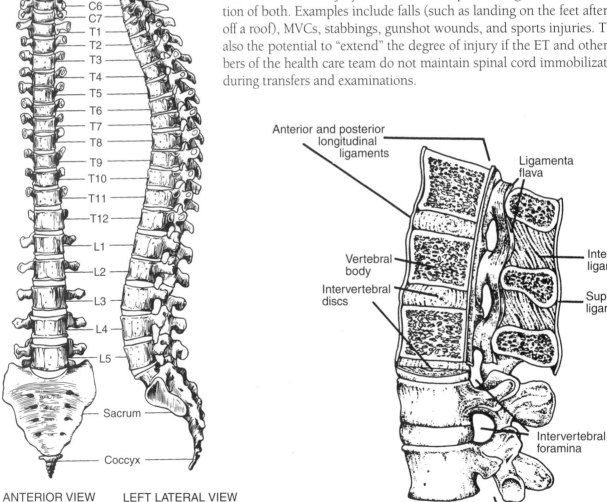

ANTERIOR VIEW   LEFT LATERAL VIEW

Figure 7-2 Vertebral Column

(Reprinted with permission from: Waxman, S., & de Groot, J. (1995). The spinal cord in situ. In *Correlative neuroanatomy* (22nd ed., p. 74). Norwalk, CT: Appleton & Lange.)

Figure 7-3 Section of the Vertebral Column

(Reprinted with permission from: Romero-Sierra, C. (1986). *Neuroanatomy: A conceptual approach*. New York: Churchill Livingstone.)

Spinal Immobilization Techniques

Patients believed to have spinal cord injuries require spinal immobilization to prevent further injury to the spinal cord. Many patients who come to the ED by ambulance already have spinal immobilization in place. The patient is lying on his or her back and unable to move. In these cases, the ET may be expected to observe the patient or assist with maintaining spinal immobilization until a physician directs the removal of the equipment. The ET also may assist in providing emotional support, monitoring the airway, and ensuring patient safety (side rails must be up).

As described earlier, maintaining a patent airway is the priority of patient care. If the spinal cord needs to be stabilized, patients should be stabilized with the cervical spine in a neutral position; in this position, the patient's spine is not flexed, extended, rotated, or placed into a lateral (side-lying) position. Recall that the spinal cord is a continuation of the brain; therefore, the head and neck are treated as a single unit to prevent motion. Cervical (neck) immobilization may be done in several ways, including: placing each hand around the base of the skull, using supportive devices on either side of the head, or using a rigid cervical collar (see **Figure 7-4**). The patient's eyes should be looking straight ahead when the head is in a neutral position. If the patient is either looking up or down, chances are the spine is in either **flexion** or **extension**. Look at the patient's ear; its opening should be lined up with the point of the shoulder when neutrally placed.

In certain conditions, placing the head and neck in the neutral position is **contraindicated**. This would occur when the position poses a threat to the patient's airway, breathing, and/or circulation.

Spinal stabilization is immobilizing the entire spine, including the cervical area. This is done with a combination of a rigid cervical collar and backboard. The patient's body and head are then secured to a backboard to prevent movement of any part of the spine. It is the role of every team member to ensure that both the head and body are secured to prevent injury.

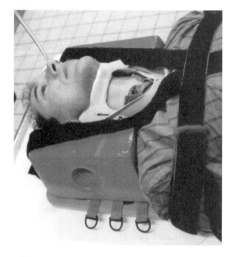

Figure 7-4 Full Cervical Spine Stabilization (Courtesy of Donna Massey, RN, MSN, CCNS.)

Cervical Collars

Cervical collars limit movement of the head and neck while reducing the loading force placed on the spine (see **Figure 7-5**). Patients who arrive at the ED with head and neck emergencies may require the application of a cervical collar. Be aware that cervical collars do not completely immobilize the head and neck but are used as a part of the total spinal cord immobilization system that includes use of the backboard and head restraint. The ET may be expected to assist with fitting and applying the correct collar to the patient. It takes practice to properly fit and apply this device. The ET usually learns this skill during orientation to the ED.

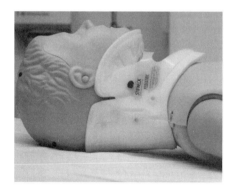

Figure 7-5 Cervical Collar Correctly Placed on Patient

Patient Assessment

Airway

Airway management is a priority in all patient care, especially when head and neck emergencies exist.

The jaw thrust maneuver is the technique of choice to open an airway in a patient with suspected neck injury. This prevents manipulation of the spinal cord, thus reducing the chances of further injury. The ET must practice this technique to become comfortable with a quick response to open the airway. (See Figure 6-1 in Chapter 6, Trauma, page 43).

Breathing

In some types of spinal cord injury, there is loss of function to the muscles that assist with the patient's ability to breathe. A patient with this type of injury will most likely be intubated and placed on a ventilator.

In other cases, the ET may be asked to assist with oxygen administration to prevent hypoxia (lack of oxygen), which is a major problem in spinal cord injury. The ET may be expected to monitor vital signs, which includes the respiratory rate. Note any breathing problems, such as breathing slowly or not at all, and report this immediately to the nurse.

Circulation

Check and document the patient's pulse frequently during the ED stay. Report any changes in circulatory status, such as decreased strength of pulse, absent pulse, cool extremities, or change in skin color.

Anticipate that the patient with a spinal cord injury may require intravenous support for medication administration and fluid replacement, if indicated. Follow the institution's policy regarding the management and care of the IV.

Disability (Neurologic Assessment)

The physician and nurse are responsible for conducting a neurologic assessment of the patient; however, the ET also may observe and report findings to the nurse. Keep in mind that maintaining a patent airway is always the priority, regardless of how severe any injury may appear. Hypoxia to the brain or spinal cord may be responsible for cell death that results in neurologic deficits. The ET may be asked to monitor the following signs and symptoms and report any changes to the nurse:

- Level of consciousness
- Orientation to person, place, time, and situation
- Memory: Long- and short-term
- Speech: Clarity and coherence
- Pupil size and response
- Motor ability
- Facial symmetry
- Sensory ability
- Skin temperature and color

A baseline examination of neurologic function is performed on all patients who come to the ED with head and neck emergencies. The frequency of these examinations is based on the patient's condition. The nurse directs the ET on how often specific observations are required. Any changes from the baseline must be reported immediately so interventions may be started to prevent further injury or loss of function.

Glasgow Coma Scale

Some hospitals require that all patients be observed and rated on a scale that quickly identifies their neurologic status. This scale is known as the

Glasgow Coma Scale (GCS) score. The maximum score is 15 and the minimum is 3 (see **Table 7-2**). When checking the GCS scores, record the *best* response to the stimulus for eye opening, verbal response, and motor response. A score of 7 or less usually indicates coma. The GCS allows the health care team to track and trend any major neurologic changes in the patient. Keep in mind that the GCS may not be accurate for patients who are intoxicated, on mind-altering drugs, <u>hypoglycemic</u>, or in <u>shock</u>.

Level of Consciousness

Level of consciousness (LOC) is an assessment of how awake and alert the patient is. To determine the level of consciousness, observe for the following:

- Is the patient awake and able to remain awake without stimulation?
- Is the patient verbal (able to speak)?
- Is the patient <u>posturing</u> (abnormal flexion or extension of arms or legs)?
- Is the patient unconscious?

Orientation

Is the patient oriented? Patients should know who they are, where they are, and the date and time. This is known as orientation to person, place, and time. Some health care providers document when the patient correctly responds to all orientation questions as "A + O × 3" (alert and oriented x 3). Some hospitals also consider orientation to the situation: Can the patient correctly identify what is happening and what caused him or her to come to the emergency department? This might be recorded as "A + O × 4." If the patient knows who he or she is, but cannot recall the date, it may be recorded as "A + O × 2 – date."

Table 7-2 Glasgow Coma Scale Score	
Areas of Response	**Points**
Best Eye Opening	
Eyes open spontaneously	4
Eyes open in response to voice	3
Eyes open in response to pain	2
No eye opening response	1
Best Verbal Response	
Oriented (e.g., to person, place, time)	5
Confused, speaks but is disoriented	4
Inappropriate, but comprehensible words	3
Incomprehensible sounds, but no words are spoken	2
None	1
Best Motor Response	
Obeys command to move	6
Localizes painful stimulus	5
Withdraws from painful stimulus	4
Flexion, abnormal decorticate posturing	3
Extension, abnormal decerebrate posturing	2
No movement or posturing	1
Total Possible Points	**3–15**
Severe Head Injury	**≤8**
Moderate Head Injury	**9–12**
Minor Head Injury	**13–15**

(Reprinted with permission from: Emergency Nurses Association. (2000). In *Trauma nursing core course (provider manual)* (5th ed., p. 56). Des Plaines, IL: Author.)

Memory

An adult patient should be able to recall his or her date of birth, past events, and recent events, such as a last meal or how he or she got to the hospital. A well child should be able to recognize a parent or caregiver, depending on the child's age. The physician performs various memory tests to identify any gaps in long- or short-term memory.

Speech

Is the patient able to speak? If so, is the speech clear and understandable? Check with the patient's caregiver to see if this is a change from normal status.

A.

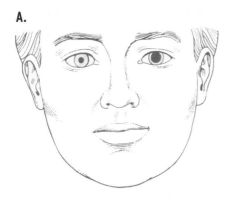

B.

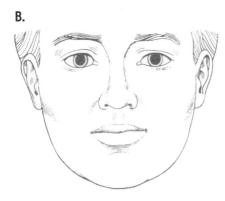

Figure 7-6 A. Pupils with One Dilated, One Normal. **B.** Both Pupils Dilated.

(Reprinted with permission from Gilboy, N. (1999). Head trauma. In Sheehy, S., Blansfield, J., Danis, D., & Gervasini, A. (Eds). *Manual of clinical trauma care: The first hour* (3rd ed., p. 190). St. Louis, MO: Mosby-Year Book.)

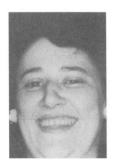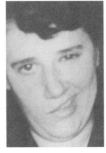

Figure 7-7 Person with a Normal Smile, and One with Facial Droop

(Reprinted with permission from Archer, W.H. (1975). *Oral and maxillofacial surgery.* (5th ed., pp. 1669, 1672). Phildelphia, PA: Saunders)

Pupil size and response

- Is the patient able to see? If so, is the vision clear and not blurred?

- Are the pupils equal in size (measured in mm)? If not, check with the patient or caregiver to determine if this is a normal condition for this patient.

- Do the pupils respond to light? Do they constrict when a light is shone into them and dilate when the room becomes darker? (See **Figure 7-6**.)

Facial Symmetry

The patient should be able to move both sides of the face equally. When smiling, does one side of the mouth droop? Is the patient able to open both eyes without a droop on one side? (See **Figure 7-7**.)

Motor Ability

- Is the patient able to move all four extremities?

- Does the patient have equal strength of both arms and legs? Test at the same time.

- Is one limb <u>flaccid</u> (the patient is unable to hold it up without help)?

- Are any of the deficiencies in motor abilities normal for this patient?

Patients who are unable to position and turn themselves need assistance in repositioning. The maximum length of time a patient may stay in one position is two hours to prevent skin injuries.

Sensory Abilities

- Does the patient have feeling in all extremities?

- Does he or she report numbness or tingling anywhere?

- Skin temperature and color may be affected by different types of trauma to the spinal cord or CNS. Abnormalities should be reported at once to the physician or nurse.

Documentation and Reporting

In some facilities, the ET may be asked to monitor the patient and record all observations, as well as report them to the nurse. Use approved medical terms for behaviors and signs and symptoms. Document them in a clear and objective manner. Compare these two statements:

- "Mr. Jones, in room 2, is very drowsy."

- "Mr. Jones, in room 2, opens only his eyes and wakes up when tapped on the shoulder for several minutes."

The second statement presents a much clearer picture of the patient's level of consciousness. Using verbage, such as "drowsy," is considered to be subjective. What one person considers drowsy may be unresponsive to another. Each hospital and facility has policies regarding documenting on the medical record. It is the ET's responsibility to be aware of the documentation process.

Radiologic Testing

With head and neck injuries, the ET must anticipate that the physician will order various types of x-rays of the head to determine the extent and severity of the injuries. X-rays of the head identify potential skull fractures. X-rays of the cervical spine are necessary in patients with neck pain related to trauma to show the position and condition of all seven cervical vertebra. The cervical collar must remain on the patient until the neck is "cleared" by the physician. Sometimes the physician orders a different view of the neck, and the ET may be asked to assist by holding the patient in the proper position to obtain this study. Always make sure to protect yourself from the x-ray beams by wearing a lead shield during the procedure.

Other types of imaging tests include computerized tomography (CT), which provide a clear picture of the anatomy of the structures and outlines soft tissues. Magnetic resonance imaging (MRI) is another test that provides an excellent picture of soft tissues and anatomic details.

Special Procedures

Logrolling

Patients with a suspected spinal cord injury should be moved only using the logrolling maneuver. The patient is assessed by the nurse or physician for neurologic deficits before and after this maneuver. One health care team member should stand and maintain head and neck stabilization during the logroll procedure. This member of the team is designated as the leader. Other team members should position themselves on the same side of the stretcher at the level of the shoulders, hips, and knees. When directed by the leader, the team works as a unit to turn or move the patient (see **Figure 7-8**).

Lumbar Puncture

The ET may be asked to assist the physician with a lumbar puncture (LP). This diagnostic test is used to measure the pressure in the spine and determine if there is blood or an infection in the cerebrospinal fluid. The physician inserts a needle between two vertebra of the spine and removes cerebrospinal fluid. The fluid pressure is measured, the color observed, and samples are sent to the laboratory for analysis. The responsibilities of the ET in assisting during this procedure may include:

- Setting up equipment in a sterile environment
- Positioning the patient. The patient must lie on his or her side in a position in which the knees are curled toward the chin. The chin is then bent forward to meet the knees (see **Figure 7-9**). The ET may need to hold the patient's knees or head to help maintain proper position for insertion of the needle. This position may affect the airway of the patient, especially with infants; therefore, close observation of the airway is required. The patient also may be in a sitting position for a lumbar puncture, as shown in **Figure 7-10**.
- Reassuring the patient during the procedure
- Labeling and transporting the specimens to the laboratory

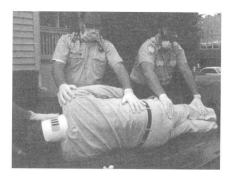

Figure 7-8 Logrolling

(Prehospital Trauma Life Support Committee of the National Association of Emergency Medical Technicians in cooperation with the Committee on Trauma of the American College of Surgeons. (1994). *PHTLS Basic and Advanced Prehospital Trauma Life Support* (3rd ed., p. 253). Philadelphia: Mosby.)

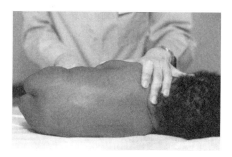

Figure 7-9 Lateral Decubitus Positioning for Lumbar Puncture

(Pediatric variations of nursing interventions. (1999). In D.L. Wong, M. Hockenberry-Eaton, D. Wilson, M.L. Winkelstein, E. Ahmann, and P. DiVito-Thomas (Eds.), *Whaley and Wong's nursing care of infants and children* (6th ed., p. 1252). Philadelphia: Harcourt Health Sciences.)

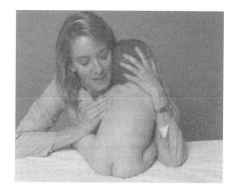

Figure 7-10 Sitting Position for Lumbar Puncture

(Pediatric variations of nursing interventions. (1999). In D.L. Wong, M. Hockenberry-Eaton, D. Wilson, M.L. Winkelstein, E. Ahmann, and P. DiVito-Thomas (Eds.), *Whaley and Wong's nursing care of infants and children* (6th ed., p. 1252). Philadelphia: Harcourt Health Sciences.)

Disorders of the Nervous System

Although there are many disorders of both the brain and spine, some are more frequently seen in the emergency care setting. Being familiar with these allows the ET to perform effectively as well as to anticipate the needs of the patient.

Increased Intracranial Pressure

With a head injury, fluids and tissues inside the skull can swell (edema) or increase in volume. When pressure becomes greater than the size of this compartment, serious problems can develop. With no place to go, the fluid and/or tissue under pressure pushes and moves nerves and other brain structures. The brain can **herniate** down through the foramen magnum, which results in death. Signs and symptoms of increased intracranial pressure include the following:

- Decreased level of consciousness
- Headache
- Nausea and vomiting
- Change in pupil size and reaction
- Seizures
- Inability to move
- Elevated blood pressure and decreasing pulse

Cerebrovascular Accident (Stroke)

A stroke is also known as a "brain attack" and may be caused by a clot in one or more of the blood vessels in the brain. The resulting lack of oxygen to the brain can temporarily or permanently damage the affected area of brain tissue. The severity of symptoms is determined by the location and amount of drainage. Common symptoms include the following:

- Numbness, weakness, or paralysis on one side of the body
- Severe headache
- Blurred or abnormal vision
- Dizziness, loss of balance
- Difficulties in speech and comprehension
- Difficulty swallowing
- Confusion

Certain types of strokes are now successfully treated if diagnosed within a certain amount of time from onset of symptoms. The ET may assist with the examination, transport of patients for a CT scan, and monitor changes in the patient's condition. The ET also may be expected to provide emotional support for the patient and family members. Patient safety is imperative, as the sudden change in physical abilities may put the patient at risk for injury.

Seizures

There are a variety of types and causes of seizures. The release of abnormal electrical energy in the brain can appear in the form of uncontrollable, abnormal body movements or a change in level of consciousness. Fever, trauma, increased intracranial pressure, low glucose (low blood sugar) and <u>**congenital**</u> disorders are some of the causes of seizures.

Maintaining the airway, followed by precautions to prevent injury resulting from uncontrollable movements, is the priority of care for the patient experiencing a seizure. This situation may be very frightening and embarrassing for the patient and the family. Some patients lose control of their bladder or bowel function during the seizure. Responsibilities for the ET may include:

- Protecting the patient's airway
- Providing patient safety
- Notifying the nurse when a seizure occurs
- Documenting or reporting to the nurse the time, duration, and specifics of the seizure activity
- Obtaining and reporting vital signs
- Providing the patient and family emotional support

Summary

The ET has a vital role in caring for patients with head and neck emergencies. Knowledge of the nervous system allows the ET to effectively support the patient, the family, and other health care team members.

Bibliography

Devinsky, O., Feldmann, E., Weinreb, H. J., & Wilterdink, J. L. (1997). *The resident's neurology book*. Philadelphia: F.A. Davis.

Shade, B., Rothenburg, M.A., Wertz, E., & Jones, S. (1997). *Mosby's EMT-Intermediate textbook*. St. Louis, MO: Mosby-Year Book.

Sheehy, S., & Lenehan, G. (1999). *Manual of emergency care* (5th ed.). St. Louis, MO: Mosby-Year Book.

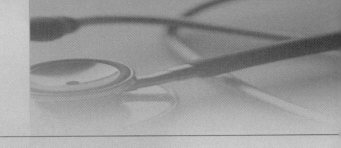

Upon completion of this module, the learner should be able to do the following:

- Describe the components of the genitourinary system.

- Discuss the role of the Emergency Technician (ET) in caring for the patient with a gastrointestinal (GI)/ genitourinary (GU) complaint.

- Identify three GI or GU emergencies the ET may encounter in the emergency department (ED).

Chapter 8

Gastrointestinal and Genitourinary Emergencies

Introduction

One of the biggest challenges the health care team faces in the ED is caring for patients with GI or GU conditions. Internal injuries resulting from blunt trauma, such as a seat belt injury to the abdomen from a motor vehicle crash or from a penetrating injury such as a stab wound, may not be identified until serious complications, such as hypovolemic shock develop. In many cases, damage to one structure may result in damage to adjacent organs or blood vessels. Medical illnesses in these body systems may take days or weeks to be recognized because some of the signs and symptoms may be very vague. The ET best serves the patient with GI or GU conditions by assisting team members with interventions, such as obtaining vital signs and specimens, providing emotional support to the patient and family members, and reporting changes in the patient's condition to the nurse.

Anatomy of the Gastrointestinal System

The GI system begins at the mouth and ends at the **anus**. Because the GI system is basically one long tube, it also is referred to as the GI tract. Ingested food passes down the GI tract and is digested into nutrients and absorbed into the circulatory system. Waste products are discarded through the anus as fecal matter.

Most of the organs of the GI system are located in the abdominal cavity (see **Figure 8-1**). The abdominal cavity extends from the diaphragm to the pelvis. A moist membrane called the peritoneum protects these organs. Within the peritoneum is the peritoneal space, which contains fluid that acts as a lubricant for the membranes.

The GI tract is divided into two major sections: The upper and lower tracts (see **Table 8-1**).

Abdominal Pain

Abdominal pain is not a diagnosis but a sign that something is wrong with the patient. When monitoring the patient's level of pain, ask for a description of the pain. Many institutions use a 1 to 10 pain scale to assess the severity of the pain, in which 1 is "no pain" and 10 is the most severe pain. Do not make suggestions unless the patient is unable to describe the pain. The physician and the nurse perform the abdominal assessment.

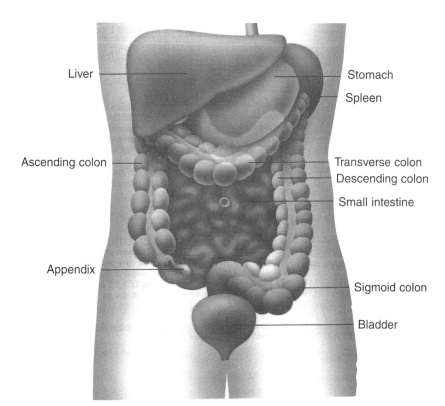

Figure 8-1 Abdominal Cavity

(Reprinted with permission from: Emergency Nurses Association. (2000). Abdominal trauma. In *Trauma nursing core course provider manual* (5th ed., p. 142). Des Plaines, IL: Author.)

Table 8-1 GI Tract: Organs and Functions

UPPER GI		LOWER GI	
Organ	Function	Organ	Function
Mouth	• Ingestion or chewing • Salivation	Small intestine • Duodenum • Jejunum • Ileum	• Chemical digestion in the duodenum; passes food into the large intestine
Pharynx	• Passage of food	Pancreas	• Enzymes break down food substances; secretes insulin, which carries glucose across cell membranes into the cell
Esophagus	• Moves food to stomach	Liver	• Bile production; metabolism of fats, carbohydrates, and proteins; produces clotting factors in the blood
Stomach	• Liquifies food into chyme with gastric enzymes	Gallbladder	• Concentrates and stores bile from the liver; bile is then released into the small intestine
		Large intestine • Ascending colon • Descending colon • Transverse colon • Sigmoid colon	• Reabsorption of fluid and electrolytes; bacteria breaks down food residue; waste products exit the body through the anus
		Spleen	• Filters blood, manufactures lymphocytes and monocytes; stores blood

Abdominal Trauma

Types of Injuries

Blunt trauma, penetrating trauma, or a combination of both may cause abdominal injuries. Blunt trauma, such as from an assault, may cause increased pressure in the abdomen, resulting in rupture of the abdominal organs. A crushing injury to the abdominal organs may result from outside forces (such as a steering wheel) pressing them against the spinal cord.

Assessing the severity of injury from blunt trauma is difficult because the ET cannot judge which organs or structures have been damaged by simply looking at the patient's abdomen. Observing a patient's condition, changes in vital signs, and the level of pain are important signs for the ET to monitor. A change in the level of consciousness may be the first indication that something is wrong. This does not mean that the patient goes from being wide awake and alert to completely unconscious for something to be wrong; instead it may occur as a change in personality or behavior. Internal bleeding may deprive the brain of oxygenated blood, which results in changes in level of consciousness.

Although patients with abdominal trauma may present with various signs and symptoms, the most common include bruising (ecchymosis) and a rigid, painful abdomen. If the patient is in a motor vehicle crash, an improperly placed seat belt may leave bruises (called a seat belt sign). Forces that are strong enough to leave this type of mark must be considered strong enough to damage underlying structures in the abdomen.

The physician may order many types of diagnostic tests for patients with abdominal trauma, ranging from simple x-rays of the abdomen to computerized tomography (CT) scans, magnetic resonance imaging (MRI), and diagnostic peritoneal lavage (DPL).

The surgeon or ED physician may perform a DPL to determine if there is internal bleeding (see **Figure 8-2**). The physician inserts a catheter into the peritoneal cavity and then attempts to withdraw (aspirate) fluid. Withdrawal of gross (bright red) blood is considered a positive finding, and the patient is taken to the operating room for exploratory surgery. If blood is not initially aspirated, a liter of warmed lactated Ringer's solution or normal saline solution is rapidly infused through the catheter. The fluid is then allowed to drain and is sent to the laboratory to check for the presence of red blood cells, bile, fecal material, white blood cells, **amylase**, or food fiber. The DPL is 98% accurate in correctly identifying abdominal bleeding.

The ET and other health care team members must remember that a nasogastric tube (NG tube) or orogastric tube (OG tube) and an indwelling urinary catheter (Foley catheter) must be inserted in the patient to avoid complications during DPL. The urinary catheter allows for continuous drainage of urine from the bladder, and the NG/OG tube decompresses the stomach, decreasing the likelihood that the catheter will accidentally hit one of these vital organs.

Penetrating trauma to the abdomen may result from a variety of mechanisms of injury, ranging from stab wounds to gunshot wounds to impalement. If a patient presents to the ED with an impaled object, DO NOT remove the object in the ED. It must be removed in the operating room. Removing an impaled object may cause the patient to hemorrhage (bleed). The ET may be asked to assist with stabilizing the object with multiple

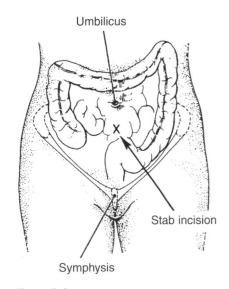

Figure 8-2 Diagnostic Peritoneal Lavage

(Reprinted with permission from: Moncure, A. (1989). Peritoneal lavage. Illustrated techniques. In *Emergency medicine scientific foundations and current practice* (3rd ed., p. 1030). Baltimore, MD: Williams & Wilkins.)

dressings and gauze to prevent movement. Depending on the part of the body affected, penetrating trauma also may cause the release of gastric acids and bacteria in the abdomen, which may lead to severe infection.

Gastrointestinal Bleeding

Bleeding may occur in either section of the GI tract. Bleeding in the upper GI tract is commonly caused by bleeding peptic ulcers, esophageal varices (from liver disease), and many other conditions. Signs and symptoms include a history of vomiting blood and black tarry stools (melena). The patient also may have a history of alcohol consumption and/or hepatitis.

Bleeding in the lower GI tract is indicated by bright red blood discharging from the large bowel and rectum. Common causes include ruptured diverticula, ulcerative colitis, tumors, ruptured hemorrhoids, cancers, and cecal ulcers.

The ET is expected to assist with the management of this patient by monitoring vital signs, assisting with NG/OG insertion, if needed, patient comfort activities, and transporting the patient to surgery or to an inpatient bed.

Anatomy of the Genitourinary System

The GU system includes the organs of reproduction together with the organs that produce urine, such as the kidneys, ureters, and bladder. The primary organs of the urinary system are the kidneys (see **Figure 8-3**). The kidneys also affect blood pressure by their secretion of an enzyme called renin. Erythropoietin, which creates red blood cells (RBCs), is also produced by the kidneys. The kidneys also produce the biologically active form of vitamin D.

Urine normally is a transparent yellow, amber, or straw color. Cloudiness indicates the presence of blood, bacteria, or drugs. Urine is composed of electrolytes (sodium, potassium, and chloride) and waste products (ammonia, urea, creatinine, uric acid). There is usually a mild odor associated with urine. The amount of urine formed by the kidneys varies by individual and depends on hormonal control and fluid intake. Men produce 800 to 2,000 milliliters (ml) of urine per day, while women generally produce 800 to 1,600 ml per day. The kidneys produce urine at a rate of 60 to 120 ml per hour. Kidney function is considered diminished or abnormal when urine output is less than 30 ml per hour in the adult, and less than 1 ml/kg/hour in the child.

The ureters bring urine from the kidneys to the bladder for storage. As the bladder fills with urine it becomes distended. The urge to void (or urinate) usually occurs

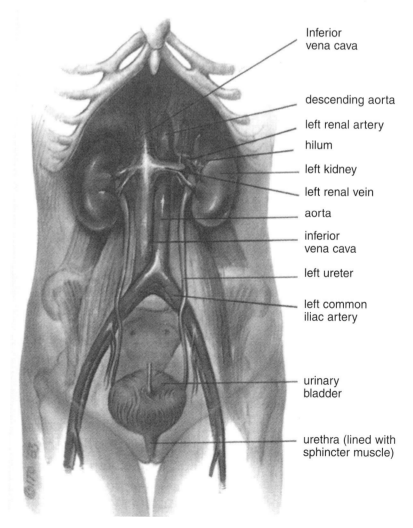

Figure 8-3 Urinary System

(Reprinted with permission from: Hegner, B.R., & Caldwell, E. (1995). The Urinary System and Common Disorders. In *Nursing assistant: A nursing process approach* (7th ed., p. 535). Albany NY: Delmar Publishers.)

- Inferior vena cava
- descending aorta
- left renal artery
- hilum
- left kidney
- left renal vein
- aorta
- inferior vena cava
- left ureter
- left common iliac artery
- urinary bladder
- urethra (lined with sphincter muscle)

when 200 to 300 ml of urine is present in the bladder. The bladder can hold up to 500 ml of urine. Urine is drained from the bladder to outside the body by the urethra. The length of the urethra varies between men and women. In women, the average length is $\frac{1}{4}$ to 1 inch, while in men it is 6 to 8 inches long. In men, the urethra also serves as a pathway for semen from the reproductive system.

In men, the prostate gland lies at the base of the bladder surrounding the urethra. The prostate is an accessory sex organ that secretes fluid into the urethra. This fluid makes up about one third of the fluid volume of the semen.

It is important to note that the urinary system is sterile and is protected by the urinary meatus and the acidity of the urine. The urinary meatus prevents the introduction of microorganisms by providing a tight closure at the distal portion of the urinary system. The acidity of the urine prevents growth of potentially dangerous bacteria; however, the acidity of the urine may cause irritation and skin breakdown when spilled on the skin. This type of skin damage may be seen in patients who are incontinent.

Infection of the Urinary System

Patients who require urinary catheterization are at high risk for development of a urinary tract infection (UTI). If left untreated a UTI can result in a serious kidney infection. Infection may result if sterile technique is not maintained during catheter insertion. The catheter serves as a conduit for microorganisms to travel through the meatus into the urinary system.

A bladder infection may change the odor and color of the urine. With a UTI, the odor of the urine becomes stronger and more offensive, the color becomes cloudy, and occasionally particles are seen in the urine. Medical treatment usually includes a prescription for an antibiotic, an antispasmotic (if patient is experiencing painful bladder spasms) along with patient education on how to prevent recurrence of the infection. If the infection goes untreated, it could lead to a more serious infection of the urinary system (i.e. pylonephritis) which would involve admitting the patient to the hospital for more agressive medical care.

Kidney Stones

Kidney stones are commonly formed from crystals of salts found in the urine. They may cause severe pain if they are large enough to block the ureter. Pain may be in the flank (back) area and may radiate to the groin. Kidney stones also can cause hematuria (blood in the urine) or pyuria (pus in the urine).

Urine samples must be strained through a special net in any patient with a potential kidney stone. Stones are then sent to the laboratory for analysis. Intravenous fluid is usually ordered to increase fluids, which may help flush the stone from the ureter. Pain from kidney stones may be quite severe, and the patient usually is given pain medication. The physician may also order an intravenous pyelogram (IVP), a radiologic exam that shows any abnormalities or blockage of the kidneys and ureters, and/or a CT scan.

Many times these stones pass through independently, especially with an increase in fluid intake. If the stone is too big to pass, the patient may need surgery.

Reproductive Organs

Conditions related to the organs of the female reproductive system that are commonly treated in the ED include infection (sexually transmitted diseases like chlamydia, syphyllis, gonorrhea), emergency childbirth, ectopic pregnancy, rape, and diagnosis of pregnancy. Men may present with infection, inflammation, trauma, and testicular torsion. The ET needs to follow the hospital's policies and procedures as well as the State Practice Act to identify his or her role in caring for a patient with this type of complaint. Cases of sexual assault (rape) are often handled by a specially trained nurse, known as a Sexual Assault Nurse Examiner (SANE) and involve obtaining legal evidence.

The ET may be asked to set up the treatment room for a pelvic examination or obtain the necessary supplies for collecting samples and transporting them to the laboratory.

In all cases, it is appropriate for the ET to be available as needed to provide comfort and emotional support to the patient.

Summary

GI and GU injuries and illnesses may be difficult to identify in the ED. Knowledge of the signs and symptoms common to these conditions, trending and tracking vital signs, and assessing pain using a pain scale helps to identify potential injuries or illnesses.

Bibliography

Emergency Nurses Association. (2000). *Trauma nursing core course (provider manual)* (5th ed.). Des Plaines, IL: Author.

Sheehy, S., & Lenehan, G. (1999). *Manual of emergency care* (5th ed.). St. Louis, MO: Mosby-Year Book.

Seidel, H.M., Ball, J.W., Dains, J.E., and Benedict, G.W. (1999). *Mosby's guide to physical examination* (4th ed.). St. Louis, MO: Mosby-Year Book.

Taylor, C., Lyllis, C., & LeMone, P. (1997). *Fundamentals of nursing: The art and science of nursing* (3rd ed.). Philadelphia: Lippincott.

Upon completion of this module, the learner should be able to do the following:

- Discuss the role of the Emergency Technician (ET) in caring for patients with musculoskeletal injuries.

- Describe how to immobilize a suspected fracture site.

- List three potential complications of musculoskeletal injury.

Chapter 9

Musculoskeletal Emergencies

Introduction

Musculoskeletal and connective tissue injuries are commonly treated in the emergency department (ED). These types of injuries are rarely life-threatening; however, without immediate and proper evaluation and treatment, these injuries can lead to lifelong disability, which can affect the psychosocial and economic status of the patient and family. When caring for a patient with a musculoskeletal injury, it is important to understand the function of a particular bone, along with which organ systems the bone may support and protect. Monitoring for potential associated organ system damage is as important as treating the presenting injury.

Anatomy of the Musculoskeletal System

The musculoskeletal system is composed of bones, joints, ligaments, tendons, cartilage, and muscles. Bones support the body by creating a frame called the skeleton (see **Figure 9-1**). This provides form and a rigid structure for muscle attachment. Muscles attach to bones by tissues called tendons. Tendons assist in movement of extremities. Bones connect to other bones by ligaments to form joints. Acting together muscles, tendons, and ligaments allow for body movement.

Bones also protect the vital organs. The brain is protected by the skull; the heart, lungs, liver and spleen are protected by the rib cage; the bladder and internal reproductive organs are contained within the bones of the pelvis. Bones also protect the marrow that is found within them; marrow contains cells involved in blood cell production.

There are primarily three types of muscle tissue within the body: voluntary, involuntary, and cardiac. The musculoskeletal system contains voluntary muscle tissue, which means that its actions are controlled by conscious thought.

Involuntary muscles are also known as smooth muscles; these are not controlled by conscious thought. Smooth muscle helps to make up the walls of internal organs, except for the heart.

Cardiac muscle is a highly specialized form of involuntary muscle tissue. When the body is at rest, the cardiac muscle will contract and relax and be ready for its next contraction in approximately 0.8 seconds.

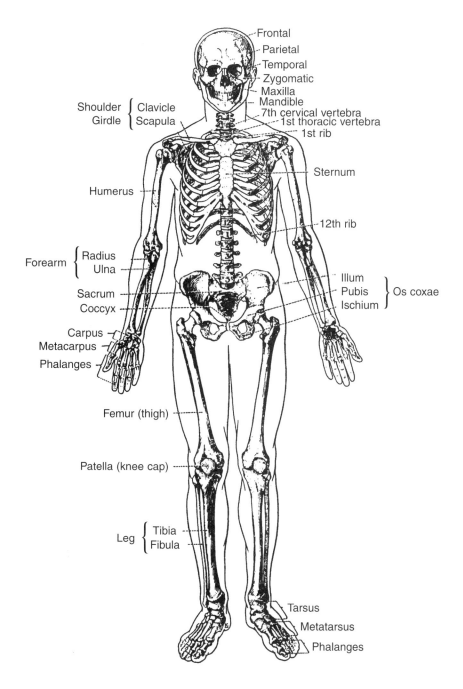

Figure 9-1 Human Skeleton

(Reprinted with permission from: WB Saunders Company. (1994). *Dorland's illustrated medical dictionary* (28th ed., Plate 44). Philadelphia: Author.)

Musculoskeletal Injury

Bones may be broken or displaced during athletic events or motor vehicle crashes, as a result of violence, or from falls (see **Figure 9-2**). Ligaments and tendons may be torn, stretched, and/or twisted. A musculoskeletal injury may result in a life- or limb-threatening injury. This may be due to a fracture of the bone or disruption of the arteries or veins. A single fracture of the femur can cause up to 1,500 ml of blood loss, and multiple fractures can lead to shock. Signs and symptoms of shock include hypotension, tachycardia, decreased level of consciousness, and cool, clammy skin. There may not be obvious areas of bleeding with fractures.

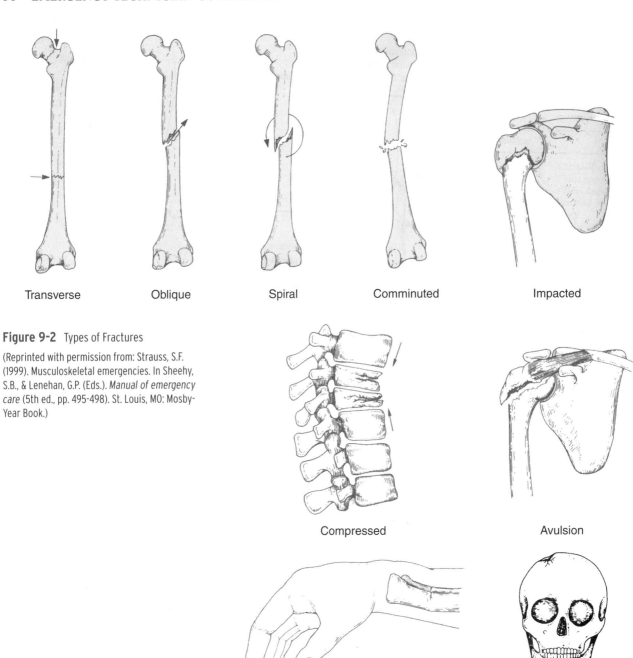

Transverse   Oblique   Spiral   Comminuted   Impacted

Compressed   Avulsion

Greenstick   Depression

Figure 9-2 Types of Fractures

(Reprinted with permission from: Strauss, S.F. (1999). Musculoskeletal emergencies. In Sheehy, S.B., & Lenehan, G.P. (Eds.). *Manual of emergency care* (5th ed., pp. 495-498). St. Louis, MO: Mosby-Year Book.)

Blood that leaks into the surrounding area of injury can lead to edema and compression of the surrounding structures. Loss of the integrity of the vessels caused by bone or joint displacement can cause ischemia or cellular death distal to the injury. With either compression or loss of vascular supply, pain increases, distal pulses become difficult to palpate, and the skin distal to the injury becomes pale, cool, and cyanotic. Nerves compressed or injured cause loss of sensation, and loss of motor and sensory function distal to the injury.

Musculoskeletal injury may be blunt or penetrating and can affect a single system injury or multiple systems. **Table 9-1** lists examples of common musculoskeletal injuries seen in the ED.

Table 9-1 Common Musculoskeletal Injuries

Injury	Description	Signs/Symptoms
Strain	• Overstretching, tearing, or overexertion of a muscle • Patient may report hearing a "snapping" sound at the time of the injury	• Weakness, numbness, localized pain made worse with movement, point tenderness, spasm, loss of muscle function, bruising (ecchymosis)
Sprain	• Stretching or tearing of a ligament	• Pain, swelling, bleeding, loss of function
Dislocation	• Displacement of a bone from its normal location in a joint	• Deformity to the extremity or joint • Decrease in movement or function
Fracture	• Break in the bone	• Muscle contractions and spasms cause shortening of the tissues around the bone causing a deformity • Pain, swelling, skin color change, loss of function, numbness, tingling
Abrasion	• Scraping of top layers of skin by a hard surface	• Pain, bleeding
Avulsion	• Full-thickness loss of skin	• Profuse bleeding, pain, pad of skin missing (i.e., finger tip pad)
Contusion	• Blood leaks into surrounding tissues without breaking the skin	• Swelling, tenderness, discoloration, bruising
Laceration	• Open wound or cut	• Bleeding, pain
Puncture wound	• Penetration of the skin by a pointed or sharp object (i.e., nail)	• Minimal bleeding, pain; high risk for infection
Amputation	• Complete separation of a limb or other body part from the rest of the body	• Profuse bleeding, pallor, obvious missing appendage, cool and clammy skin

Care of the Patient with Musculoskeletal Injury

Patients who present with a musculoskeletal injury also may have additional injuries. It is important for the ET to remember that even though the injured limb may be very evident, there may be underlying injuries that need to be attended to first. Start with the ABCs (airway, breathing, and circulation). If the patient does not have a patent airway and is not able to breathe, it does not matter that the leg is broken. Frequently monitor the vital signs of a patient with multiple trauma or multiple fractures. Once the immediate life-threatening injuries are treated, then assist with caring for the rest of the patient's injuries.

Immobilize the affected limb above and below the suspected fracture site. Immobilization protects the limb from further injury to the bone, vessels and nerves. Next, elevate the extremity to the level of the heart. If there is an impaled object, stabilize and protect the extremity until the object can be removed by the physician (or in surgery). Applying ice packs to the affected extremity provides some pain relief and decreases the swelling. Remember, never apply ice directly to the skin because it causes tissue damage; instead, wrap it in a towel or use specially designed ice packs that come with coverings. Initially, cover any open wounds with a sterile dressing until the nurse directs you to clean or dress the wound. Anticipate that this patient will also need one or more x-rays taken of the injured limb.

In addition to these general interventions, the ET may be asked to observe the patient's neurovascular status. Always compare the injured side to the uninjured side to identify differences. If both the injured and uninjured feet are cool to the touch, it does not necessarily mean there is a problem. This could be normal for the patient; however, if the injured foot is cool and pale, but the uninjured foot is warm and pink, the nurse must be notified immediately so corrective action may be taken. Observation should include the five Ps:

- Pain—intensity, location, throbbing, burning
- Pallor—color of the extremity
- Pulses—presence, strength
- Paresthesia—numbness, tingling, or altered sensation
- Paralysis—inability to move the affected limb

During the course of the patient's stay in the ED, report any changes you may notice.

While musculoskeletal injuries are rarely life-threatening, potentially life-threatening complications may occur if these injuries are not properly identified and treated. Complications include the following:

- Infection
- Loss of function or mobility
- Hemorrhage (bone fragments pierce underlying organs or structures)
- Loss of sensation from nerve damage (permanent or temporary)
- Chronic pain
- **Arthritis**
- Disturbances in growth, especially in children if the growth plate is damaged
- **Compartment syndrome** (A potentially limb threatening emergency where increased pressure in the limb from a variety of sources such as swelling, bleeding or a cast; causes compression of nerves and muscles.)
- **Fat embolus** (A mass (thrombus) of fat that can migrate through the blood stream causing blockage of blood vessels.)
- Shock (A syndrome resulting from inadequate blood flow to tissues and cells in the body leading to a decrease in the supply of oxygen and nutrients.)
- Death

Impaired Mobility

Injury to bones, muscles, tendons, ligaments, and cartilage can limit a patient's mobility. Devices such as crutches, canes, casts, and splints are used to mobilize or immobilize the affected area. Patient teaching is pro-

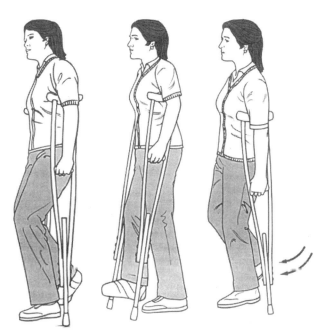

Figure 9-3 Crutch Walking Gait

(Reprinted with permission from: Proehl, J. A., & Jones, L. M. (1997). *Mosby's emergency department patient teaching guides* (p. I-7). St. Louis, MO: Mosby-Year Book.)

vided regarding the use of these devices. It is very important to test the patient's ability to use these devices correctly before discharge from the ED. Inappropriate use may result in injury.

Crutches

Crutches and canes must be correctly fitted to the patient (see **Figure 9-3**).

Many hospitals have physical therapists available to help fit the patient for crutches and teach crutch-walking techniques. Check with the facility to find out what your role is regarding this intervention.

Splints, Casts, and Wraps

Some injured extremities need to be immobilized, either with a splint or a cast, until an orthopedic surgeon can follow-up with the patient. Some minor musculoskeletal injuries require application of a compression bandage (Ace® wrap). The role of the ET is to assemble the necessary equipment, assist the physician or nurse with application of the device, and provide emotional support for the patient and/or family members. Many casts are now fitted using little, if any, water, and are molded to a specific position that supports and immobilizes the limb. Many splints now have Velcro® attachments that make it easy to adjust and readjust the splint for comfort and function. Most hospitals will provide the ET with training specific to the materials used during orientation to the ED.

Re-evaluate the neurovascular status of the extremity distal to the injury after application of the cast or splint. The color of the nail beds should remain pink, the skin should be warm, and there should be no change or decrease in sensation.

Tips for Measuring Crutches

1. Have the patient lie on the stretcher wearing his or her shoe on the unaffected foot.

2. Measure the distance from the anterior fold of the armpit (axilla) down to the heel and then add 2 inches to that number. That is the length of the crutches needed. Some crutches come presized. Ask the patient how tall he or she is and select the appropriately packaged crutches.

3. Have the patient stand upright to adjust the handgrips on the crutches. Proper length allows the hand to reach the grips with a slight bend to the elbow.

4. Remind the patient not to use crutches while wearing socks or high heels on the uninjured foot; this puts the patient at increased risk for falling and further injury.

5. Instruct the patient to support the body weight with the hands and arms, not with the armpit when crutch walking. This could cause nerve damage to that area as well as pain and bruising.

6. The nurse will cover additional patient education information such as how to climb up and go down stairs and whether it is safe to drive a car with the patient's particular injury.

Summary

When caring for patients with a musculoskeletal injury, the ET must be aware of the function of the injured part, as well as the associated structures that may also be affected. Frequent observation of the area and prompt reporting of any changes to the nurse helps to prevent further damage or loss of function. In this role, the ET is crucial to the outcome of patient care.

Bibliography

Seidel, H.M., Ball, J.W., Dains, J.E., and Benedict, G.W. (1999). *Mosby's guide to physical examination* (4th ed.). St. Louis, MO: Mosby-Year Book.

Sheehy, S., & Lenehan, G. (1999). *Manual of emergency care* (5th ed.). St. Louis, MO: Mosby-Year Book.

Taylor, C., Lyllis, C., & LeMone, P. (1997). *Fundamentals of nursing: The art and science of nursing care* (3rd ed.). Philadelphia: Lippincott.

Thomas, C.L. (Ed.) (1997). *Tabor's cyclopedic medical dictionary*. Philadelphia: F.A. Davis.

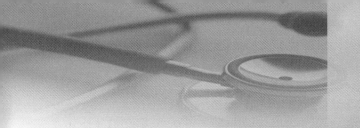

Surface Trauma

Upon completion of this module, the learner should be able to do the following:

- Discuss the basic principles of wound care.

- Identify the four burn classifications.

- Describe the role of the Emergency Technician (ET) in caring for the patient with burns.

Introduction

Skin or soft-tissue injuries are commonly seen in the emergency department (ED). Even though these types of injuries are seldom life-threatening, the blood vessels or nerves may be damaged at the same time, leaving the patient at risk for complications such as shock or loss of limb. Burn injuries, which may range from mild to severe, are another type of soft-tissue injury often treated by the ED health care team.

The Skin

The skin is part of the integumentary system, which also includes the layers directly under the skin, the hair, glands in the skin, and the nails (see **Figure 10-1**). The outer layer of the skin is called the epidermis, which contains no blood vessels or nerves.

The epidermis has several layers and gives the skin its color. Below the epidermis is the dermis. This layer contains blood vessels, nerves, sweat

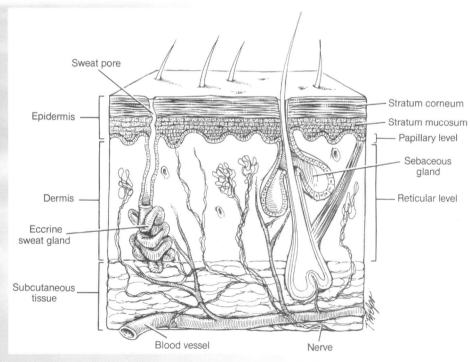

Figure 10-1 Anatomy of the Skin

(Reprinted with permission from: Whitney, J. D. (1994). Wound healing. In Cardona, V. D., Hurn, P. D., Mason, P.J. B., Scanlon, A. M., & Veise-Berry, S. W. (Eds.). *Trauma nursing from resuscitation through rehabilitation* (2nd ed., p. 267). Philadelphia: Saunders.)

glands, oil glands, and hair follicles. The dermis contains nerve endings that are involved with the senses of touch, cold, heat, and pain. Below the dermis are layers of fat and soft tissue called the subcutaneous layers. The skin has many functions:

- Protects the underlying organs by acting as a shock absorber
- Regulates body temperature
- Carries sensations from the environment to the brain
- Eliminates waste products such as salt (in sweat) and carbon dioxide
- Helps to maintain water and electrolyte balance
- Produces and absorbs vitamin D from sunlight

Types of Wounds

Many different types of surface wounds are seen in the ED (**Table 10-1**). Wounds may be described as superficial or deep. A superficial wound involves capillary bleeding only, and the depth of the wound does not extend past the dermis. With these wounds, sutures are not needed to control bleeding or for wound repair. A deep wound may involve blood vessels and nerves and extends beyond the dermis. This type of wound typically requires some wound closure by the physician.

Wound Repair

Before a wound can be repaired, it must be irrigated and/or debrided (when the dead tissues are cleared away). The ET may be expected to assemble necessary equipment and assist the physician with the wound repair. Several methods may be used, including suturing, staples, adhesive closures, or "gluing." Special glue and adhesive closure strips may be used for minor or superficial lacerations. The edges of the wound are brought together using adhesive strips or glue. No anesthetic is needed for this type

Table 10-1 Common Wounds Seen in the ED

Type of Wound	Description
Abrasion	Scraping of the top layers of skin by a hard surface
Amputation	Complete separation of a limb or other body part from the rest of the body
Avulsion	Full-thickness loss of skin
Contusion	Blood leaks into surrounding tissues without breaking skin
Incision	Surgical laceration or wound with smooth edges
Laceration	Open wound or cut
Puncture	Penetration of the skin by a pointed or sharp object (i.e., nail)

of repair, which is an advantage especially when caring for young children.

Staples may be used for deeper lacerations to the scalp, torso, and extremities. This is a quick way to close the wound and is often used to control bleeding in trauma patients who need immediate intervention. The ET needs to gather the following equipment for this procedure:

- A wound stapler

- Wound cleaning equipment (sterile gauze, saline solution, and povidine iodine solution)

- An anesthetic

- Antibiotic ointment and bandaging supplies

Suturing is a commonly used for wound closure (see **Figure 10-2**). Most hospitals have prepackaged suture trays with most of the necessary sterile supplies assembled. This tray must be opened using a sterile technique to prevent contaminating the instruments. There are two small cups in the tray. One is filled with normal saline solution, and the other, povidine iodine solution. Providine iodine solution must never be used on the area of an injured tissue; it is used only to cleanse the skin around the injured area, as it can damage the tissue cells. Suture scissors, needle holders, and forceps are in the t ray, as are syringes, needles, gauze pads, and sterile towels. The physician will need sterile gloves, suture material, and a local anesthetic (usually 1% or 2% lidocaine). If the wound needs to be irrigated prior to repair by the physician, a larger catheter-tip syringe, an 18-gauge IV catheter, sterile basin, and normal saline solution are used. For wounds that contain dirt or other foreign bodies embedded in the wound, a surgical brush may be used for cleaning. Some hospitals have specific equipment designed for irrigation.

Assemble the suturing equipment on the bedside table on the side closest to the injury. If the patient is a child, some type of restraint or additional bedsheets may be needed to keep the child from moving too much during the procedure, or the child may need to be sedated. Children are very often frightened by the experience and should remain with a caregiver as much as possible during the procedure. Do not restrain a child until the physician is ready to begin. It may be necessary for the ET to hold the affected area during the repair to limit movement. This is especially true with head or facial lacerations and extremity injuries.

After the procedure is finished, gently clean any blood from around the area of the wound and pat it dry with a sterile 4 × 4 gauze. The physician may instruct the nurse to apply an antibiotic ointment on the wound before bandaging. If a dressing is ordered, place a sterile mesh gauze dressing containing a water-soluble lubricant on top of the wound to prevent sticking. Then cover the wound with gauze and secure in place.

Complications may occur during the wound-healing process, including allergic reaction from anesthetics, cleaning solution, suture material, or antibiotics; excessive bleeding; swelling; infection; inflammation; and scarring.

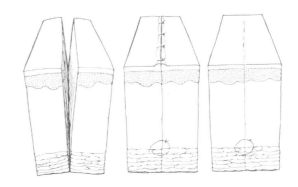

Figure 10-2 Wound Healing Suturing by Primary Closure.

(Reprinted with permission from: Whitney, J. D. (1994). Wound healing. In Cardona, V. D., Hurn, P. D., Mason, P.J. B., Scanlon, A. M., & Veise-Berry, S. W. (Ed.). *Trauma nursing from resuscitation through rehabilitation* (2nd ed., p. 284). Philadelphia: Saunders.)

Table 10-2 Burn Classification

Type of Burn	Description	Example
Superficial partial-thickness or first-degree burn	Involves the epidermis; pain and redness without blistering	Sunburn
Partial-thickness or second-degree burn	Involves the epidermis and part of the dermis; very painful, blisters and mottled (spotted) skin	Scalding injury from hot water
Full-thickness or third-degree burn	Involves the epidermis, the entire dermis, and into the subcutaneous tissue; nerve endings are destroyed so there is no pain. Skin is charred black, or areas are dry and white.	Severe frostbite

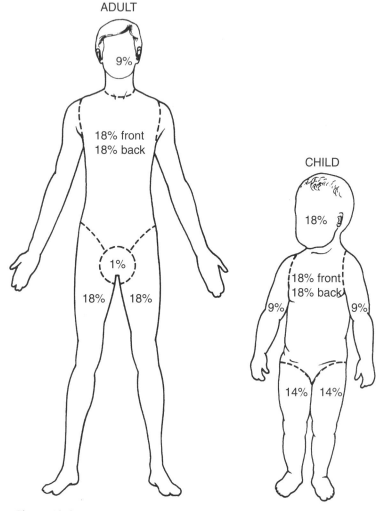

Figure 10-3 The Rule of Nines

(Reprinted with permission from: Emergency Nurses Association. (2000). Burn trauma. In *Trauma nursing core course (provider manual)* (5th ed., p. 219). Des Plaines, IL: Author.)

Burns

There are three major types of burns: thermal, chemical, and electrical (see **Table 10-2**). Patients exposed to thermal, chemical, or electrical energy need immediate attention to stop the burning process and prevent further injury. Thermal burns are the most common type and are caused by flame, flash, scald, or contact with hot objects. One complication of exposure to thermal energy is inhalation injury. This type of injury can occur when the respiratory tract is exposed to intense heat, poisonous chemicals, or smoke. Prompt attention to the airway must always be given to the patient with an inhalation injury. Chemical burns are caused by direct contact with caustic agents such as acids or alkali. Electrical burns are caused by exposure to electrical current, such as AC or DC electricity or lightning and are much more difficult to assess because the injury may be internal. Electrical burns may have an entrance and exit site visible on the skin.

Burns that require care in a burn center include partial- or full-thickness burns greater than 20% of total body surface area, burns on the face, hands, feet or **perineum**, burns in the very young and the very old, and full-thickness burns greater than 5% of total body surface area.

The percentage of the body burned can be determined by using the rule of nines evaluation tool (see **Figure 10-3**).

Burn Care

Burn care in the ED focuses on stopping the burning process and maintaining the ABCs—airway, breathing, and circulation. If the face and/or chest area is burned, the lungs are most likely affected as well. It is important to have oxygen delivery devices at the bedside. Patients are placed on 100% oxygen using a nonrebreather mask. The patient also must be placed on a pulse oximeter to monitor oxygen saturation levels (**Caution:** Patients who have carbon monoxide poisoning will not have accurate readings.) A cardiac monitor may be indicated if the burn is extensive or if the patient has electrical burns.

Remove all jewelry from the patient's wrists and fingers because body parts may swell in response to the burn. Jewelry may need to be cut off if swelling has already developed because jewelry could possibly block blood flow to distal areas.

The ET must have equipment available and supplies ready for burn care, including sterile basins, sterile towels, sterile bottles of cooled and room temperature normal saline solution, sterile gloves, masks, and sterile gowns. Some institutions may have burn packs, which contain sterile sheets, blankets, and towels. Sterility is essential because the skin has lost its barrier protection and the risk of infection has increased. Sterile gloves are necessary for contact with all burns in which skin is no longer intact, and gowns and masks should be worn to care for all patients with moderate to major burns.

Initially, sterile towels soaked in cooled saline solution may be used on the burn area to stop the burning process, depending on the body surface area burned. Because of the risk of hypothermia, there is debate over whether cooled saline solution should be used; however, this may not be recommended if the total body surface area burned exceeds 10%. It is important to check the institution's policy and procedure manual regarding this practice. Burn patients can quickly become chilled due to the loss of skin and secondary injury. After the cooling process is completed, replace the wet bedding and linens with dry sterile sheets and blankets in order to maintain a more normal body temperature.

Many burns require a dressing before the patient is admitted, transferred to a burn unit, or discharged. The nurse may direct the ET to apply antibacterial burn cream and a dressing; however, if no burn cream is applied, the burn should be covered with a mesh gauze that contains a water-soluble lubricant to prevent sticking. Next, a bulky dressing, such as 4 × 4 gauze sponges approximately ¹/₂-inch thick, is applied to absorb drainage. Secure bulky dressings with a semi-elastic gauze, and wrap extremities distal to proximal. It is important to wrap the patient's hands in a position of function (i.e., fingers slightly flexed with the thumb drawn away from the palm by putting a roll of gauze in the palm to support the position). Equally important, wrap fingers and toes separately to allow for movement, leaving the tips exposed to check circulation.

Common complications of burns include infection, sepsis, blood loss, nerve and/or blood vessel damage, loss of function of an extremity, and death.

Summary

Skin and soft-tissue injuries, though seldom life-threatening, may result in shock or loss of function. Understanding the possible complications and principles of wound and burn care will help ensure that ED patients have the best possible outcomes.

Bibliography

Collier, I. C., Heitkemper, M., & Lewis, S. M. (1996). *Medical surgical nursing: Assessment and management of clinical problems* (4th ed.). St. Louis, MO: Mosby-Year Book.

Kidd, P., & Stuart, P. (1996). *Mosby's emergency nursing reference.* St. Louis, MO: Mosby-Year Book.

Porter, W. (1996). *Porter's pocket guide to critical care* (5th ed.). Chicago: Porter and Associates.

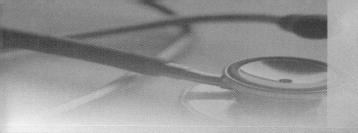

Upon completion of this module, the learner should be able to do the following:

- Discuss the role of the Emergency Technician (ET) in caring for a patient with injuries or illnesses to the eyes, ears, nose, and throat.

- Explain how to perform a visual acuity test.

- Describe the steps involved in eye irrigation.

- Discuss methods to control epistaxis.

Eyes, Ears, Nose and Throat Emergencies

Introduction

Problems associated with the eyes, ears, nose, and throat (EENT) are rarely life-threatening unless the airway is affected; however, any impairment or loss of function to these senses may be very traumatic as well as life altering to the patient. As with any other condition, the patient's airway, breathing, and circulation (ABCs) must be assessed before focusing on specific injuries.

The Eye

Parts of the Eye (see Figure 11-1)

Iris	The colored part of the eye; muscular control over the amount of light that enters the eye by changing the size of the pupil
Pupil	The black center of the eye; constricts and dilates in response to light; controlled by cranial nerves. Certain drugs affect pupil response.
Cornea	Covers the iris.
Sclera	The white part of the eye (around the iris); covered by a thin membrane called the conjunctiva.
Aqueous Humor	Watery fluid in the anterior chamber of the eye (in front of the lens); fluid made continuously and excess drained.
Vitreous Humor	Gel-like fluid in the posterior chamber of the eye (behind the lens); not produced continuously; leakage affects the shape and function of the eye.

Visual Acuity Testing

A visual acuity test must be performed for patients who present with eye complaints. The patient is asked to identify pictures or letters on a Snellen™ chart placed at a specific distance (usually 20 feet) from the patient (see **Figure 11-2**). Numbers on the side of the chart denote how far the patient sees compared to a 20-foot scale. One eye is tested at a time. Cover the eye not being tested with a hand or some other type of barrier. Test vision of the affected eye first, then the uninjured eye, and then both together. Ask

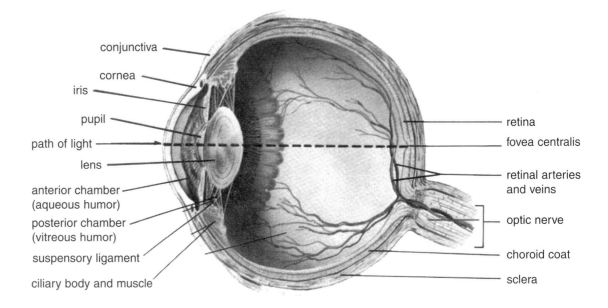

Figure 11-1 Cross Section and Frontal Diagram of the Eye

(Reprinted with permission from: Hegner, B., & Caldwell, E. (1995). Basic anatomy and physiology. In *Nursing assistant: A nursing process approach* (7th ed., p. 73). Albany, NY: Delmar Publishers.)

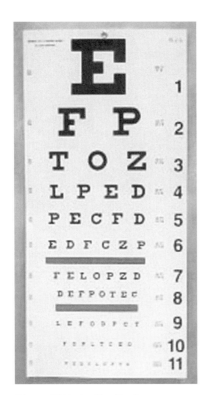

Figure 11-2 Snellen Chart

(Reprinted with permission from: Smallwood, M. (1999). Assessing visual acuity. In Proehl, J. A. (Ed.). *Emergency nursing procedures* (2nd ed., p. 499). Philadelphia: Saunders.)

the patient to read the letters on each line of the chart until he or she begins to make errors. Record the last line the patient read correctly. If the patient reads the 20/50 line, he or she sees objects at 20 feet that the normal eye sees at 50 feet. All three readings are recorded in the patient's record using the appropriate medical abbreviations: OD refers to right eye, OS refers to left eye, and OU is both eyes. If the patient missed one letter in a line when using the right eye, it may be charted as OD: 20/50 −1. Also, note whether the patient wears corrective lenses (e.g., glasses, contact lenses) and if he or she was wearing them at the time of the visual acuity examination.

Eye Injuries

The structures of the eye are very delicate and easily injured. Treatment must be started quickly to prevent permanent damage, especially with chemical splashes.

Foreign Bodies

Foreign bodies in the eye are very painful. The foreign body may be visible, or the physician may use a slit lamp or Wood's light to find it. A slit lamp acts as a microscope for the examination of the eye. A Wood's light is a cobalt blue light that detects any irregularity in the cornea after **fluorescein dye** is put in the eye. If a foreign body is not imbedded in the eye or is lying on the surface, it may be removed by irrigation. If a foreign body is imbedded, it must be removed by the physician and may require surgery.

Penetrating Trauma

Never try to remove a penetrating object (e.g., fish hook) from an eye. The ET may be asked to assist with stabilization to prevent further movement without putting pressure on the globe (eyeball)(see **Figure 11-3**). Since both eyes move symmetrically, the uninjured eye should be covered with an eye patch to limit eye movement.

Corneal Abrasions or Injuries

A corneal abrasion is a scratch to the surface of the cornea by a foreign body, such as from a piece of metal or wood. Individuals who wear contact lenses also are at risk for corneal abrasions. These injuries are exceedingly painful because the surface of the cornea is scratched and the corneal nerves are exposed. There is a lot of tearing, and the patient may report sensitivity to light. With these injuries, the physician will instill fluorescein dye because any abrasion to the eye is more visible when using an ultraviolet light. The foreign body may still be in the eye at this time. Treatment typically is an antibiotic ointment and an eye patch applied to the injured eye.

Overexposure to sunlight, tanning booths, and arc welding without protective eye wear may cause surface burns to the cornea. These burns are very painful and make the eyes very sensitive to light. However, the pain usually does not develop until a few hours after the exposure. Allow a patient with possible surface burns to sit in a darkened room while waiting to be examined.

Chemical Burns

Chemical splashes to the eye are very dangerous and may lead to loss of vision (see **Figure 11-4**). Quick action is needed to prevent permanent damage. The damage from a chemical burn depends on the amount and concentration of the chemical and the length of time the chemical is in contact with the eye. Usually, alkaline chemicals cause more damage than acidic chemicals and require longer time to irrigate. Patient outcomes are usually better if an initial eyewash was done at home or at the job site before the patient arrived to the ED. The nurse or physician may instill anesthetic eye drops prior to the examination to decrease the pain. The ET then may irrigate the affected eye(s) with normal saline solution. Irrigation continues until the **pH** of the eye reaches 7.0. If extensive and prolonged irrigation is necessary, it is helpful to use a continuous irrigation device (such as Morgan Lens™). Use of this device is more comfortable for the patient, and once the device is inserted into the eye, it is virtually a hands-free operation, allowing the ET to perform other duties.

Procedure for Irrigating the Eye

- Wash hands.

- Insert appropriate tubing into irrigating solution and clear the line of air.

- The nurse or physician instills anesthetic eye drops to make the procedure easier for the patient to tolerate.

- Instruct the patient to lie flat.

- Pad around the patient's head with towels, or give the patient an emesis basin to hold along the side of the face to catch irrigating solution runoff. The head of the bed may be positioned so the patient may hang his or her head into the sink to allow runoff to flow directly into the sink.

- Apply examination gloves.

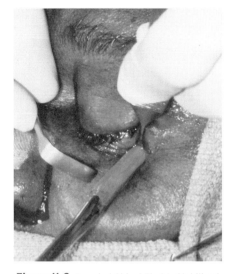

Figure 11-3 Impaled Object That Is Stabilized

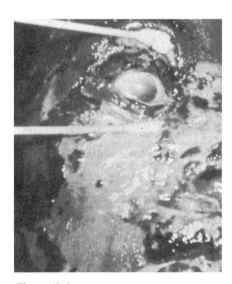

Figure 11-4 Chemical Burn

(Reprinted with permission from: Deutsch, T. A., & Feller D. B. (1985). In *Paton and Goldberg's management of ocular injuries* (p. 95). Philadelphia: Saunders.)

- Gently rinse the eyelids with irrigating solution so exterior contamination does not flow into the patient's eyes during irrigation.

- Hold the patient's eye open with one hand or ask the patient to assist. To obtain a better grip, hold the eye open with 4 × 4 gauze. Ask the patient to look up as the solution flows onto the eye.

- Always let the fluid flow from the inside of the eye to the outside so runoff fluid does not contaminate the opposite uninjured eye.

- Instruct the patient to look in another direction as fluid continues to irrigate the eye and to blink in an attempt to dislodge a foreign body, if appropriate.

- Continue irrigation until the prescribed amount of solution has been used, or the pH of the eye is 7.0.

- Document the amount and type of solution used and any effect on the patient.

To irrigate the eye using the Morgan Lens™, follow the same procedure as outlined above. In addition, attach the Morgan Lens™ to the end of the tubing and clear the line of air. The physician or nurse instills anesthetic eyedrops. The Morgan Lens™ is placed on the eye by slipping it under the upper eyelid and then gently pulling back the lower lid to insert the bottom portion of the lens cup. Release the eyelid so it covers the lens to hold it over the eye. Tape the irrigation tubing to the patient's forehead and open the IV clamp to provide continuous flow. Remember to pad around the patient's face with towels to soak up irrigation solution (see **Figure 11-5**).

Figure 11-5 Eye Irrigation & Morgan Lens

(Reprinted with permission from: Mortan, Inc., (1996). Instructional chart for Morgan lens. Copyright 1996 by Mortan, Inc., Missoula, MT.)

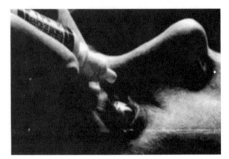

Instill topical anesthetic if available.

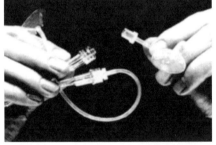

Attach Morgan Lens® Delivery Set, I.V., or syringe using solution and rate of choice; **start flow.**

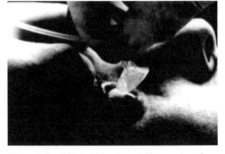

Have patient look down, insert Morgan Lens® under upper lid. Have patient look up, retract lower lid, drop lens in place.

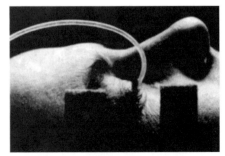

Release the lower lid over Morgan Lens® and adjust flow. Tape tubing to patient's forehead to prevent accidental lens removal. **Do not run dry.**

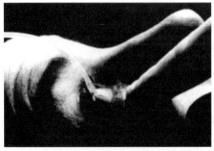

Removal: Continue flow, have patient look up, retract lower lid—hold position.

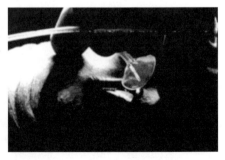

Slide Morgan Lens® out, **terminate flow.**

To remove the lens, instruct the patient to look up, while gently pulling down on the lower lid and removing the bottom portion of the lens. Then, ask the patient to look down, and pull back the upper lid to remove the lens. Document the amount and type of solution used and any effect the procedure had on the patient.

Blunt Trauma

Assaults, motor vehicle crashes, and sports injuries may cause blunt trauma to the eye and the surrounding structures. <u>Periorbital</u> edema and ecchymosis can indicate a soft-tissue injury, as well as injury to the eye or the facial bones.

Blow-out Fracture

The orbital bones that make up the socket of the eye are very thin and fragile. If the patient receives a blow to the eye, these bones may break causing a blow-out fracture of the orbit. Muscles and surrounding nerves of the eye may become trapped in the fracture site which may lead to permanent disability. If this occurs, the eye may have a sunken appearance, and the patient may experience double vision and limited up and down movement of the eye (see **Figure 11-6**). These symptoms may disappear as the swelling decreases. If not, surgery may be required.

Patients should be cautioned not to blow their nose or hold their breath or bear down as it may cause nerve entrapment and permanent visual disabilities.

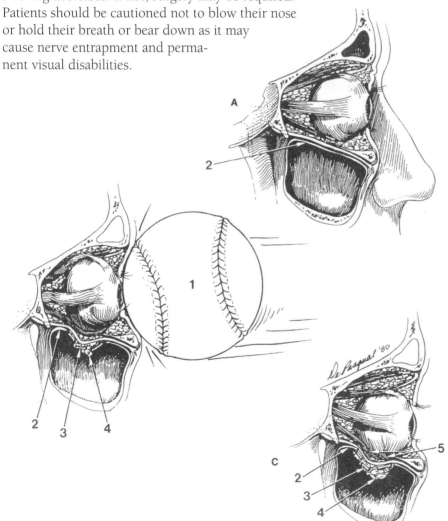

Figure 11-6 Blow-out Fracture

(Reprinted with permission from: Gerlock, A.J., McBride, K. L., & Sinn, D.P. (1981). In: *Clinical and radiographic interpretation of facial fractures.* Philadelphia: Saunders.)

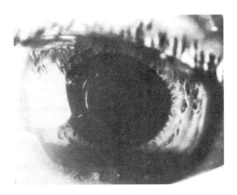

Figure 11-7 A hyphema

(Reprinted with permission from: Deutsch, T. A. & Feller D. B. (1985). In: *Paton and Goldberg's management of ocular injuries* (p. 188). Philadelphia: Saunders.)

Hyphema

A hyphema may occur as a result of blunt trauma to the eye. With a hyphema, blood partially or completely fills the anterior chamber of the eye (see **Figure 11-7**). The optic nerve is damaged with the prolonged pressure in the eye caused by **glaucoma**. Therefore, any patient with a hyphema requires consultation with the **ophthalmologist**. While waiting for this consult, place the patient in a quiet area, cover the eye with a patch to avoid any further trauma, and elevate the head of the bed to decrease intraocular pressure. The patient should avoid any activities that increase intraocular pressure, such as straining, coughing, or blowing the nose. If the patient complains of nausea, the physician may direct the nurse to give an **antiemetic** to prevent vomiting which could increase intraocular eye pressure, and cause permanent damage to the eye.

Retinal Detachment

A retinal detachment occurs when the two layers of the retina separate. This may be caused by trauma but also may be caused by retinal degeneration. Retinal detachment more often affects people over 40 years of age, particularly those with diabetes.

The patient reports seeing flashes of light, even when the eyes are closed, and may see showers of black dots in the peripheral vision. The patient may describe the condition as a "curtain" pulled over his or her sight. Any patient with a retinal detachment requires an immediate ophthalmology consult. Both eyes are patched to decrease eye movement, and the patient is placed on bedrest while awaiting surgery.

The Ear

The ear is divided into three areas: External, middle, and inner ear (see **Figure 11-8**).

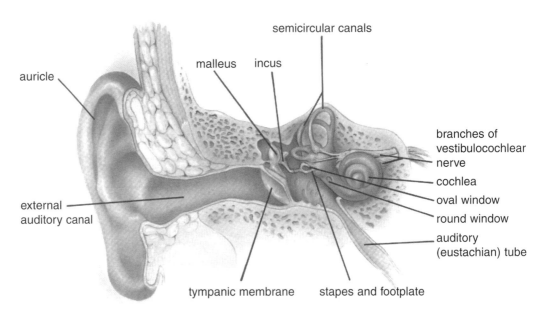

Figure 11-8 Diagram of the Ear with Reference Points

(Reprinted with permission from: Hegner, B., & Caldwell, E. (1995). Basic anatomy and physiology. In: *Nursing assistant: A nursing process approach* (7th ed., p. 75). Albany, NY: Delmar Publishers)

Parts of the Ear

External Ear

- Auricle or pinna: Captures sound waves and directs them into the ear

- Ear canal: Conducts sound waves to ear

- The tympanic membrane, or eardrum: Separates the external ear from the middle ear

Middle Ear

- Malleus, incus, and stapes: Three small bones or ossicles that transmit sound.

- Air-filled cavity that connects to the nasopharynx by the eustachian tube.

Inner Ear

- Vestibule: Affects balance and equilibrium

- Cochlea: The hearing center

- Semicircular canals: Affect balance and equilibrium

Injuries to the Ear

Injuries to the external ear frequently result from assaults. Direct pressure and ice packs are applied to control bleeding and swelling. Blood in the ear canal may be caused by injury to the external ear or a cerebrospinal fluid leak, which indicates a skull fracture.

The tympanic membrane may become perforated with the insertion of an object, such as a cotton tip applicator. It may rupture during an explosion, direct blow to the ear, or as a result of an ear infection. Most of the time the tympanic membrane heals on its own, but a physician must examine the patient.

Foreign Bodies

People often insert objects into their ears, especially children. Sometimes, the object is not discovered until a discharge is noticed coming from the ear. Insects, such as cockroaches, also may crawl or fly into ears, which causes great distress to the patient, especially if the insect is still alive and moving. A lidocaine solution may be instilled into the ear to anesthetize the insect or to cause it to crawl out. Sometimes mineral oil is placed in the ear to drown the insect to make removal easier. The ET may be asked to hold a child while the physician removes the foreign body.

The Nose

The nose is the organ of smell as well as a passageway for air to enter the respiratory system (see **Figure 11-9**). The nose filters, moistens, and controls the temperature of the air before it passes into the lungs. The nose also plays a part in speech and taste. Infants breathe primarily through their noses and may experience difficulty in breathing if the nasal passages are blocked.

The olfactory membranes are located in the roof of the nasal cavity, just beneath the bridge of the nose; these membranes contain the receptors for smell.

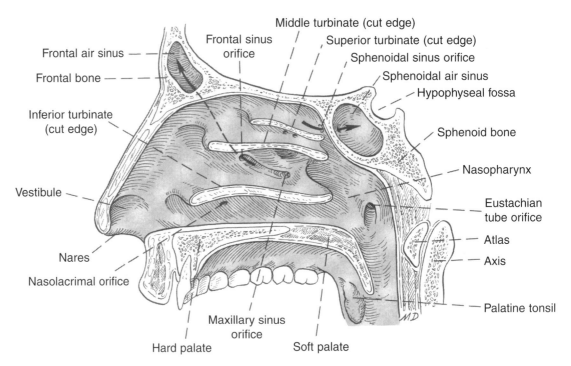

Figure 11-9 Cross Section of the Nose and Nasal Cavities

(Reprinted with permission from: Nield, M. (1993). Structure and function of the respiratory system. In: Black, J. M., & Jacobs, E. M. (Eds.). *Luckmann and Sorensen's medical-surgical nursing: A psychophysiologic approach* (4th ed., p. 901). Philadelphia: Saunders.)

The sinus cavities connect to the nasal cavities by small channels. The sinuses are named for the skull bones under which they lie: The frontal sinus, ethmoid sinus, sphenoid sinus, and maxillary sinus. The sinuses are lined with mucous membranes and secrete mucus into the nasal cavities.

Epistaxis

<u>Epistaxis</u>, or nosebleed, may occur in the anterior or posterior section of the nose. Anterior bleeding occurs in any age group and is typically caused by dry air, allergies, nose picking, or trauma. Initial treatment is pinching the fleshy part of the nose for at least 10 minutes. Ice packs also may be applied to the nose to decrease bleeding and swelling. Once the bleeding has stopped, the patient must be cautioned not to blow his or her nose as this may start the bleeding again.

If the bleeding does not stop with these measures, the physician may try to cauterize the area of bleeding with silver nitrate sticks. The nose also may be packed with specially treated tampons to help control the bleeding. Patients may be discharged with this gauze packing in place and be instructed to return in two to five days for follow-up care.

Posterior bleeding usually occurs in older adults as a result of atherosclerosis of the nasal vessels, liver disease, or from medications such as anticoagulants. Posterior nosebleeds also may be caused by congenital clotting disorders. It is controversial as to whether high blood pressure causes nosebleeds or if it just increases the bleeding once it starts. Only 10% of nosebleeds are posterior bleeds.

Posterior bleeding cannot be stopped by pinching the nose, cautery, or by gauze packing because the sites of bleeding are not accessible. The patient must be in a sitting position to be able to easily spit out any blood that drips down the back of the throat. Blood is very irritating to the stomach and may cause the patient to vomit.

There are various balloon tamponade devices on the market to control posterior nasal bleeding (see **Figure 11-10**). A nasal balloon or catheter is inserted into the posterior nare. The balloon is inflated to apply pressure to the bleeding areas. Traction is placed on the balloon. Petroleum gauze packing is inserted into the nose to surround the tube. Hospitalization usually is necessary because of the potential for the device to become dislodged and cause airway obstruction.

If there has been a lot of bleeding, the patient may need IV fluid replacement. With severe blood loss, the patient may need a blood transfusion. Medications may be given to decrease the blood pressure if the patient is hypertensive. Epistaxis may be very frightening to the patient, and the ET needs to maintain a calm, reassuring manner when caring for these patients.

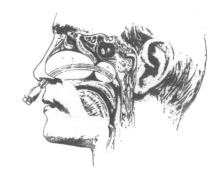

Figure 11-10 Nasal Balloon Packing
(Reprinted with permission from: Medtronic Xomed, Jacksonville, FL.)

Blunt Trauma

Blunt trauma to the nose may occur from assaults, motor vehicle crashes, sports injuries, or falls. Ice is applied to the nose to decrease swelling and help stop bleeding. Gentle pressure is applied to the fleshy part of the nose. Often the bleeding stops without further intervention. Patients with nasal fractures may or may not have surgery depending on the severity and need for repair.

Foreign Bodies

Children may insert foreign bodies (e.g., toys, food) into the nose. The first indication that parents or caregivers may have of the problem is the presence of a foul-smelling drainage or bleeding from the nose. Removal of the foreign body may require sedation or surgery if the child is unable to cooperate. The ET may be asked to hold the child while the physician removes the foreign body.

The Throat

The throat, or pharynx, is the passage that leads to the digestive and respiratory systems.

Infection

The mucous membranes of the throat are very vascular and are often the site of inflammation and infection. Patients often present to the ED with a bacterial or viral infection of the throat.

Hemorrhage

Hemorrhage is a serious postoperative complication of a tonsillectomy. Severe bleeding is a true emergency because of the potential for airway compromise and shock from blood loss.

Penetrating Trauma

Objects, such as lollipop sticks and pencils, may become imbedded in the throat of an individual if they should fall on them. Never try to remove any penetrating object. The ET may assist with stabilization of the object until the physician can safely remove it. Puncture wounds to the throat may pose serious risk of damaging major blood vessels in the throat.

Foreign Bodies

Foreign bodies, such as food, may become lodged in the throat. Respiratory arrest may develop if the foreign body completely obstructs the airway. Abdominal thrusts (Heimlich maneuver) may remove the obstruction. If this is not successful, the physician may try to remove it with specially designed forceps.

A conscious, breathing patient may be given medication to relax the esophagus to allow the obstruction to pass. If other methods do not work, surgery may be needed to remove the obstruction.

Summary

The ET plays an assistant role in the management of EENT emergencies. Patients with these conditions usually are anxious about the potential for loss of one of their senses. A calm, reassuring approach helps to relieve the patient's anxiety and fears.

Bibliography

Agur, A. (1991). *Grant's atlas of anatomy.* Baltimore, MD: Williams and Wilkins.

Bates, B. (1992). *A guide to physical examination and history taking* (5th ed.). Philadelphia: Lippincott.

Bressler, K., & Shelton, C. (1993). Ear foreign body removal: A review of 98 consecutive cases. *Laryngoscope,* 103(4 Pt 1), 367–370.

Henry, M. (1997). *EMT prehospital care* (2nd ed.). Philadelphia: Saunders.

Nettina, S. (2000). *The Lippincott manual of nursing practice* (7th ed.). Philadelphia: Lippincott.

Rosen, P. (1998). *Emergency medicine concepts and clinical practice* (4th ed.). St. Louis, MO: Mosby-Year Book.

Sanders, M. (1994). *Mosby's paramedic textbook.* St. Louis, MO: Mosby-Year Book.

Williams, P.L. (Ed.). (1999). *Gray's anatomy* (38th edition). Edinburgh, NY: Churchill Livingstone.

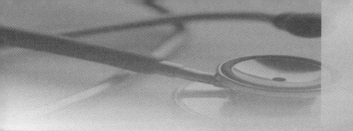

Psychological and Emotional Issues

Upon completion of this module, the learner should be able to:

- Identify the causes of stress.

- Identify five characteristics of the patient at risk for suicide.

- Discuss proper restraining techniques.

Introduction

Psychosocial issues have a direct influence on the health of individuals and how they perceive the care that they receive. They also impact the ability of the health care team to provide care to their patients. Understanding the complexity of psychosocial issues and how to deal effectively with their components is an important aspect in patient care delivery.

Stress

Stress occurs as a reaction to emotional and physical conditions in the environment, and it may occur from real or imagined sources. A certain amount of stress is considered healthy and allows individuals to adapt to changes in their lives by learning and growing from the experience. Stress may be caused by many factors.

Personal life stress may be caused by one or more of the following:

- Financial problems

- Demands of family and loved ones

- Personal or family illness or death of a loved one

- Pressure for time to get things done

- School

- Marriage, divorce, or separation

- Buying or selling a house

- Vacation

- Moving

Work stress may be caused by one or more of the following:

- Noise

- Staffing problems, busy shifts, or rotating shifts

- Changes in systems, procedures, and policies

- Computer or technology breakdowns

- Abusive or demanding patients and visitors

- Poor relationships with coworkers

- Critically ill or injured patients
- Problems with equipment
- Morale issues
- Job insecurity
- Lack of confidence or knowledge in skill performance

The emergency department (ED) can be an overwhelming place for patients and their families. The unfamiliar surroundings and fear of illness or injury also may cause stress. Other causes of stress for patients and their families in the ED include any one of the following:

- Pain
- Fear of disfigurement or disability
- Possible loss of work time
- Loss of control or loss of ability to cope
- Commitments at home
- Lack of communication from staff
- Cost of the ED visit
- Fear of death
- Noise in the environment

Reaction to stress depends on perception, past experience, and the ability to deal with the situation. At times, perceptions and past experiences do not provide the coping skills needed to deal with the stress. At this point stress becomes overwhelming and interferes with the ability to make decisions.

Behavioral and Psychiatric Emergencies

Behavioral emergencies require different skills than medical or trauma care. Patience, compassion, and understanding are some of the most important qualities needed in the care of these patients. Intervention must be timely in order to prevent a crisis situation.

Behavioral emergencies may occur for reasons other than a psychiatric problem. Other causes for altered mental status and behavioral changes include substance abuse, hypoxia, head injury, stroke, brain tumor, shock, renal or liver failure, infectious illnesses, hypoglycemia or hyperglycemia, and seizure.

Selected Psychiatric Emergencies

Anxiety

Mild anxiety may make a person more alert and better able to deal with problems; however, when anxiety becomes overwhelming, fears may be out of proportion. Patients may have panic attacks and may be unable to cope with normal events. Signs and symptoms of severe anxiety may imitate other potentially life-threatening conditions, such as a heart attack. Other signs and symptoms include the following:

- Hyperventilation (breathing too fast)
- Shortness of breath
- Chest pain

- Heart palpitations; fluttering sensation in the chest; fast pulse
- Choking sensation or difficulty swallowing
- Dizziness
- Trembling
- Sweating
- Urinary frequency
- Diarrhea

Care of the patient with severe anxiety includes a calm bedside manner and not leaving the patient alone. It is helpful if a family member stays with the patient during his or her evaluation if this does not increase the patient's anxiety level. Pay attention to the patient's fears, and do not disregard his or her concerns. The physician may order medication to help decrease the patient's anxiety level.

Mania

Mania is a state of extreme excitement. Many patients who demonstrate this behavior have bipolar disorder, a condition in which they fluctuate between mania and depression. Mania also may be caused by drug abuse. Signs and symptoms of mania include excessive happiness, a fast speech pattern, talking a lot, delusions of grandeur, and perhaps a recent history of spending sprees. A calm, quiet, direct approach helps define boundaries and acceptable behavior for these patients. Decreasing the stimulation in their environment by turning down the lights and moving them to a quiet area may help as well.

Depression

Depression is an abnormal sadness that is out of proportion to the event or situation. Depression may be a symptom of a mental disorder or may be the primary diagnosis. A patient with depression is typically physically inactive, has a lack of desire to socialize, has feelings of worthlessness, loss of self-esteem, and thoughts of self-injury or destruction. Specific signs and symptoms include the following:

- Loss of appetite
- Decreased libido (sex drive)
- Difficulty sleeping or excessive sleeping
- Constipation
- Decreased energy
- Feelings of guilt

It may take many attempts to convince a patient to open up and talk about his or her feelings. Therefore, it is best to have the same person provide care rather than a variety of people interacting with the patient.. Depressed patients may have a negative self-concept and wish to harm themselves. Ask all patients who are depressed if they are suicidal. Asking the question does not put the idea into their head.

Suicide

Patients who are suicidal require immediate attention. Do not assume that a patient will not commit suicide because he or she came to the ED seeking help for suicidal thoughts. It is difficult to distinguish between a suicide gesture and a suicide attempt. Any gesture should be taken seriously, and the patient should be evaluated by a mental health professional.

Patients at greater risk for suicide include those who have tried to commit suicide in the past. Men tend to be more successful completing suicide, while women attempt suicide more often. People over age 55, or those who have a lack of religious ties, live alone, are isolated, withdrawn, or who may lack satisfying work are at a higher risk for attempting suicide. In addition, a family history of suicide, substance abuse, chronic debilitating illness, recent loss of a loved one, or changes in finances increase the risk for suicide. A patient with a formed suicide plan and means available (i.e., owns a gun), or a history of mental illness such as depression, paranoid schizophrenia, or other psychosis must be placed on suicide precautions. Never leave a suicidal person alone!

A search of patient belongings must be done upon admission to the ED treatment room. Remove all clothing and place the patient in a hospital gown. In one real-life situation, a piece of glass was found in socks that were left on a patient. Many hospitals have a special treatment room for patients who are suicidal or having a psychiatric emergency.

Potentially dangerous equipment that the patient could use for self-harm or to harm others should be removed from the room. Follow the institution's protocol for the handling of weapons.

Psychosis

Psychotic patients experience major distortions of reality. They may be disoriented and unable to function. They may have hallucinations, bizarre thoughts, or may hear voices telling them to do something. They may be withdrawn or **catatonic**. Paranoia or phobias are common, as is the potential for violence or suicide.

A psychotic patient must be assessed for the potential for violence. This potential increases if there is a history of past episodes of violence, the patient assumes a threatening pose or posture, or has loud, obscene, and erratic speech patterns.

Identify yourself when approaching the psychotic patient. Be calm and courteous without being too familiar. To prevent agitation, do not make any sudden moves or respond to any of their statements in anger. Speak in normal tones, and do not whisper with relatives or others outside the patient's room because this may increase their feelings of persecution (paranoia).

Critical Incidents

A critical incident is defined as any event that overwhelms the normal coping abilities of a person. The emotional response to these incidents is so intense it impairs the person's ability to function.

Team members in the ED are involved with tragic events that may interfere with their ability to continue to provide care. Team members may feel guilt or despair because they were unable to save a life. What might be considered a "critical event" for the emergency technician (ET) may not be for another coworker, depending on the ability to cope and past experiences with this type of situation.

A number of critical events are commonly seen in the ED, as follows:

- Unsuccessful resuscitations
- Death of a child
- Caring for someone the staff knows personally
- Multiple victims or a disaster
- Highly publicized events (i.e., shooting of a police officer)
- Acts of violence
- Situations that remind the caregivers of a person or occurrence in their own lives

Critical Incident Stress Debriefing

Critical incident stress debriefing (CISD) is a process used to help ED and rescue personnel deal with these overwhelming situations. During a CISD, mental health professionals or trained peers meet with everyone involved with caring for the patient, including prehospital personnel. This meeting usually occurs within the first two days of the event. The purpose of the CISD is not to find fault, place blame on anyone, or identify mistakes. Rather, it is an opportunity for everyone to discuss the event in a supportive, confidential environment so they may explore their feelings about the event rather than trying to cope alone. A discussion in this type of supportive environment helps staff get back to work and continue to take care of patients in a safe and competent manner as well as successfully deal with the stress the event may have had on their personal lives.

Postmortem Care

The ET may be responsible for preparing a patient's body for viewing by the family in the ED. Make sure that all blood and secretions are removed from the patient's face and hands before allowing the family to come into the treatment room. If possible, lay one arm on top of a clean top sheet so the family is able to touch the patient. Do not remove or touch any IV lines, endotracheal tubes, chest tubes, or other equipment until directed by the nurse.

If the funeral home does not come to the ED to pick up the body right away, the body needs to be transported to the hospital morgue. It is very important that there is an identification band or some other identification in place prior to transport. Exact procedures vary with each institution. A morgue stretcher, which is specially designed to hide the body from the public's view, may be used. Give valuables to the family, and document what was given to whom and when. Before giving any of the patient's belongings or valuables to anyone, check with the nurse to make sure that the patient is not involved in a police investigation. In this case, the belongings or valuables may be considered evidence.

Restraints

Restraints are commonly used on children in the ED to prevent movement during a procedure, such as suturing; however, a patient who is violent or suicidal may need to be restrained for the safety of the staff as well as the patient. Restraints provide control for patients when they no longer have control of themselves. The nurse or physician explains the reasons for physical restraint to patients prior to restraining them, if possible. If other calming techniques have failed and the decision is made to restrain a patient, there must be a clear plan. Stay at least an arm's length away until help arrives. At least four people are needed, one for each limb, to safely restrain a patient. Be aware of the surroundings and remove potentially harmful objects from the room. During orientation, the ET learns the physical skills, as well as the related policies, to safely restrain a patient.

Common principles of applying restraints include the following:

- Restrain the patient to the bed, not to the side rails

- Attach restraints firmly to all four extremities

- Ensure that the restraints are not too tight by making sure you can insert two fingers between the restraint and the extremity

- Check the circulation of the patient at least every 30 minutes for leather restraints and every 60 minutes for soft or Velcro restraints, or according to your hospital's restraint protocol.

Summary

When caring for patients with psychiatric illnesses, keep the following principles in mind:

- Be nonjudgmental

- Use good listening skills

- Allow the patient some control

- Be flexible, not rigid

- Stay calm

- Watch what is said and how it is said, including body language

- Identify one person to communicate with the patient

The ET is more effective when he or she understands the emotional and psychological events a patient may be experiencing. Gaining confidence in dealing with patients who are grieving or experiencing behavioral emergencies takes practice. Taking care of your own mental health is an important step in ensuring that you can function in the role of an ET.

Bibliography

Emergency Nurses Association. (1998). The pediatric patient. In *Emergency nursing pediatric course* (2nd ed., pp. 21–38). Park Ridge, IL: Author.

McSwain, N. (1997). *The basic EMT.* St. Louis, MO: Mosby-Year Book.

Sanders, M. (2000). *Mosby's paramedic textbook* (2nd ed.). St. Louis, MO: Mosby.

Stoy, W. (1996). *Mosby's EMT basic textbook.* St. Louis, MO: Mosby-Year Book.

Chapter 13

Safety and Violence Prevention

Introduction

The ED setting tends to be busy, noisy, and unfamiliar to patients and visitors. This environment may put patients at further risk for injury, as well as increase the potential for violence. It is important to identify patients at risk for injury to themselves and to others to provide a safe environment in the ED.

Patient Safety

Falls are considered one of the most common incidents in the ED that result in patient injury. Falls occur for many reasons. A patient may be confused and try to climb off the stretcher; a sudden change in position may cause a loss of balance that produces changes in vision or depth perception leading to a fall. The best way to prevent a patient from falling is to identify patients who are at risk for falls. Patients that may be at risk for falling include the following:

- Elderly patients

- Pediatric patients, especially if not under the direct supervision of a caregiver

- Patients who have been given medications, especially for pain

- Patients who are confused or intoxicated

- Patients who have impaired mobility, such as paralysis or injury to the legs

- Patients in restraints

Following general safety measures not only helps protect those patients who are at risk for falls, but makes the ED a safer place. There are a number of general safety rules to follow in the ED, as stated below.

- Floors are clean and dry without spills or clutter.

- Walkways are clear.

- Equipment is kept close to the wall.

- Stretchers with patients on them are kept in the lowest position with the side rails up and brakes in the locked position.

- Sharp or dangerous objects are kept out of the patient's reach.

- Patients at risk for falling, while walking or on a stretcher, must not be left unattended.

- Any broken or malfunctioning equipment must be reported and removed from use immediately.

Staff Safety Issues

Violent acts are on the rise in health care facilities. The Emergency Technician (ET) should be aware of the security measures in the institution and his or her role in assisting others to provide for the safety of the staff and patients. It is also important for the ET to recognize the circumstances that may precipitate violence, and what can be done to prevent its occurrence or escalation of an event.

The ED is open 24 hours a day, seven days a week and it is often the only entrance to the hospital after business hours. Because of this unrestricted access, ED staff must be alert for anything or anyone that might jeopardize their safety.

Safety measures vary among institutions, depending on their location and history of violence. Safety measures work only when used consistently and properly. Examples of safety measures used by an ED may include any of the following:

- Full-time security guards or police stationed in the ED

- Metal detectors

- Key cards or access codes to gain entrance to the ED (see **Figure 13-1**)

- Alarm systems or panic buttons

- Guard dogs

- Surveillance cameras (see **Figure 13-2**)

- Direct telephone lines to local police departments

- Special code words announced on the overhead pager that identifies a dangerous situation and calls for help

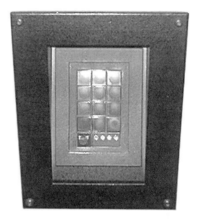

Figure 13-1 Key Pad Access

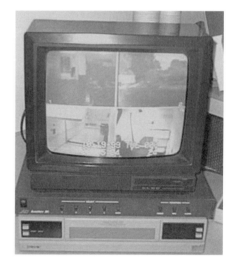

Figure 13-2 Security Camera

Triggers for Violence

Acts of violence are often predictable. The ET should be alert for specific triggers that increase the potential for violence in either the patient or the people who accompany the patient to the hospital. They include the following:

- Fear and anxiety about their pain, injury, or illness

- Fear and anxiety about a loved one who is a patient. This is especially true if a visitor has been waiting and has not received information or has received incorrect information about the patient.

- A history of violent behavior

- A history of alcohol or drug abuse

The violent patient generally has a history of violence. He or she tends to have poor impulse control and low self-esteem. If you ignore or belittle individuals with this type of behavior, it may serve to inflame an already stressful situation. The ET must speak firmly, with respect, as well as be aware of body language (nonverbal communication).

Predictors of Violent Behavior

Individuals who become violent exhibit behaviors that will alert the ET that an act of violence may occur, if measures to intervene appropriately are not taken. Examples of these behaviors are listed below:

- Speaking loudly and quickly
- Pacing, and repetitive behaviors, such as foot tapping
- Tense body language, such as fist clenching, gritting teeth, facial expressions
- Use of violent gestures
- Use of threatening words or foul language
- Drug or alcohol intoxication, especially if the patient is in withdrawal

Patients with psychiatric disorders may have a difficult time understanding their surroundings and events. Patients experiencing paranoia may feel trapped and wish to escape—at any cost. A noisy environment, forceful mannerisms, and sudden movements may predispose these psychiatric patients to act out. When interacting with this type of patient, create a quiet environment with few distractions. Use simple words in short sentences, and allow time for the patient to express his or her needs.

It is important to remember that medical conditions may also predispose a person to violence. Hypoxia or hypoglycemia may make a patient combative until that condition is reversed. Other examples include head injuries, chemical imbalances, and dementia.

The Assault Cycle

The assault cycle has a predictable pattern identifying what happens before, during, and after an assault. Understanding how a person moves through the assault cycle and the type of interventions needed for each stage of the cycle helps the ET in violence prevention. The stages of the assault cycle are listed below (see also **Table 13-1** for more information):

- Triggering event
- Escalation phase ("fight or flight")
- Assault phase
- Recovery phase
- Postcrisis phase

Understanding the assault cycle will help to decrease the potential for violence, but there are times when a violent act may occur even when the ET or staff members have responded appropriately. A number of techniques can be used to deal with a potentially violent person, as listed below.

- Always approach the person calmly.
- Treat all patients and co-workers with respect and dignity.
- Never be alone with a potentially violent person in an isolated place.
- Always leave yourself an exit from the area.

Table 13-1 Stages of the Assault Cycle

Stage	Definition	Example	Interventions
Triggering Event	• Associated with a loss or perceived loss	• Being a patient in the ED with an injury of any type may be a triggering event. • A family member who is admitted for chest pain	• Assist the patient in identifying healthy coping strategies and support systems.
Escalation Phase	• Acting out in response to the triggering event; the patient reacts to the perceived event by "fight or flight"	• A patient curled up in the corner of a room who is unwilling to communicate is an example of "flight." • A patient who becomes agitated, whiny, aggressive, manipulative, or non-communicative is an example of "fight."	• Empathetic communication may be helpful. Saying "I see you are angry. Would you like to tell me about it?" begins to build a relationship with the patient. • Use simple words and short sentences; set limits.
Assault Phase	• If the escalation phase is allowed to continue	• The assault may be verbal or physical.	• Assault is an unlawful act and must be reported in all cases. • It may be appropriate to restrain the person.
Recovery Phase	• May last for moments or days	• The patient continues to be very vulnerable during this phase, and if the perceived threat returns, violence may recur.	• Frequent communication is necessary during this phase.
Postcrisis Phase	• The time period after the violent act has occurred	• The patient feels remorseful for his or her actions and wants forgiveness. • The patient feels depressed and may withdraw.	• Re-establishing open communication with this individual is crucial at this time.

- Leave doors open when talking with a potentially violent person.
- Do not touch or move toward a potentially violent person.
- If threatened, firmly inform the person that violence is not tolerated.
- If the violent behavior escalates, leave the area and follow the hospital's policy for dealing with the violent person.

It is important to understand that even if the ET recognizes and intervenes early, there are times when violence will still occur. If violence does occur, the goal is to protect yourself, the patient, and others from injury. Do not try and deal with a violent patient alone. Call for help. If assaulted, turn the care of the patient over to another health care worker.

Summary

The ET plays a vital role in keeping the environment safe in the ED. Observation and awareness of the surroundings and the behaviors of individuals will help alert the ET of the potential for violence, allowing for early intervention or prevention of the event.

Bibliography

Coastal Video Communication Corp. (1997). *Health care violence: Be a part of the cure.*

Kitt, S., Selfridge-Thomas, J., Proehl, J.A., & Kaiser, J. (1995). *Emergency Nursing: A physiologic and clinical perspective* (2nd ed.). Philadelphia: Saunders.

McQuillan, K.A., Von Rueden, K.T., Hartsock, R.L., Flynn, M.B., and Whalen, E. (2002). *Trauma nursing from resuscitation through rehabilitation* (3rd ed.). Philadelphia: Saunders.

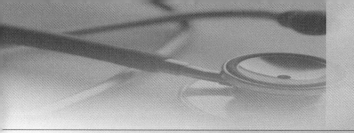

Legal Issues

Upon completion of this module, the learner should be able to:

- Describe responsibilities and accountabilities associated with the delegation process.

- Define the four elements of professional negligence.

- List six intentional torts and practices and how to prevent them from occurring.

- Name five types of patient consent.

- Describe the importance of accurate record keeping and patient confidentiality.

Introduction

The law is a dynamic and ever-changing part of our lives. Many of the laws under which the Emergency Technician (ET) practices are controlled by the state or municipality. Specific legal questions or other specific information regarding legal issues should be referred to the institution's legal counsel. For institution-specific situations, institutional and departmental policy manuals should be utilized for guidance.

Within the emergency department (ED) setting, the ET faces many different types of situations that have legal significance. Familiarity with these issues and individual scope of practice is very important when performing duties and providing patient care. This knowledge also serves to protect the patient, the ET, and other staff members.

Delegation and Responsibilities

The American legal system traditionally has held that any health care provider is accountable for his or her own actions. Therefore, all health care providers must understand the importance of maintaining knowledge, skills, and practice competencies.

Delegation of responsibilities to unlicensed assistive personnel (UAP) remains a controversial topic in health care. Both the emergency nurse and the ET have a responsibility to know the limitations of their scope of practice. While nurses may delegate certain tasks to the ET, they may not delegate the primary nursing functions of assessment, evaluation, and judgment. A nurse who delegates improperly may be liable for any negative outcomes resulting from the ET's care. The ET also has a responsibility to inform the nurse or supervisor when improper delegation has occurred.

Under the theory of respondeat superior, which means to "let the master answer," the hospital may be liable for the errors of its employees. In other words, the employer is responsible for the wrongful acts of its employees. Employers are almost automatically included as an additional defendant in a lawsuit. An employer may try to argue that it is not responsible if an employee is not acting "within the scope and course of their employment." Exceeding the job description and performing duties not authorized by the institution's policy is not covered by the employer's malpractice insurance; therefore, the ET must understand his or her job description and the skills that are included within the context of the job.

Professional Negligence

Health care professionals today should be aware of the risks for litigation based on care they rendered to a patient. A lawsuit for professional negligence is commonly called malpractice.

There are four elements that the plaintiff (the party suing) needs to prove to successfully pursue a case of professional negligence: duty, breach of duty, causation, and damages. These terms are defined below in the context of the ET.

Duty

Duty is concerned with whether the ET had a responsibility to provide care to the patient. Usually there is no duty to care if an individual is not on-the-job; however, the ET does have an obligation to care for the patient when working in the ED.

Breach of Duty

Breach of duty is failure to provide the type of care that would be provided by a reasonably prudent person with the same or similar medical training. The patient would argue that the care provided was substandard or fell below the standard of care. The breach can be accomplished by commission, which is performing an act (or in this case, patient care) that a reasonable person would not, such as putting a cast on the wrong extremity. A breach also can occur by omission, which is a failure to act; an example is failing to provide crutch-walking instructions prior to sending a patient home using crutches for the first time.

The issue of whether a breach has occurred usually is established by expert testimony. A health care professional with the same or similar training is hired to testify as to the "standard of care" that should be given to the patient under the same or similar circumstances. The standard for the ET is that of a reasonably prudent Emergency Technician with the same amount of experience working under similar conditions.

Causation

Causation is the relationship between actions and the injury. This is where the party who is initiating the lawsuit must prove that "but for" the ET's actions the patient would not have been harmed. Causation is often the most difficult element of negligence to prove. An example of causation is failure to raise a patient side rail as the immediate cause of the patient's broken hip, because the hip was broken as a result of the patient falling off a gurney. In legal terms, the ET's failure to raise the side rails was the foreseeable cause of the patient's injury.

Damages

In order to successfully bring a lawsuit, there has to be an actual injury, such as pain, suffering, mental anguish, hospital and medical expenses, loss of future earning capacity, and/or wrongful death. Monetary damages are sought to compensate the patient or family for the injuries sustained.

Intentional Torts

Intentional torts may occur when the ET is working in direct contact with patients. These include abandonment, assault, battery, false imprisonment, and invasion of privacy, libel, and slander. It is important to be aware of these issues, as they may result in litigation and, ultimately, liability.

Abandonment

Abandonment is defined as premature termination of patient care or release of the patient to a provider who cannot provide care at an equal or greater level. An example of abandonment is transport of a patient to a nursing unit and then giving the patient report to the unit secretary rather than to the receiving nurse. If the patient's condition deteriorates, the secretary will not be held liable since he or she has no responsibility to provide patient care. The ET may be held liable for "abandoning" the care of that patient. To avoid problems with this issue the ET must remain with the patient once patient care is initiated until the patient is safely transferred to a care provider with equal or greater medical knowledge.

Assault

Assault occurs when a health care provider (or any individual) causes fear or threat of unauthorized touching. It does not matter whether the actual touching ever occurs. To avoid problems with this issue, the ET should advise the patient what intended care or treatment is about to be given, and obtain the patient's consent before ever touching the patient.

Battery

Battery is the touching or treating of the patient without consent. To avoid committing battery, obtain patient's consent before touching him or her.

False Imprisonment

False imprisonment is the intentional and unjustifiable detention of a patient. It is most often an issue when restraints are used improperly. Physical restraints may be appropriate when they are used in the best interest of the patient—to protect the patient and the staff from harm. To avoid problems with this issue, use only reasonable force when applying restraints. As a protective measure, document the medical necessity of the restraints and try to obtain consent.

Invasion of Privacy

Invasion of privacy occurs when an ET is aware of private or personal information about the patient and in some fashion, reveals this information to a person or persons who are not directly involved in the care of the patient. The ET may be liable if this information, even if accurate, conveys a false impression or subjects the patient to public ridicule. To avoid problems with this issue, be cautious in communicating any type of patient information. Do not discuss private patient information with unauthorized individuals. Avoid sharing confidential information about the patient with friends or family members.

Libel

Libel is injury into a person's character, name, or reputation by false or malicious written accusations. To avoid problems with this issue, be cautious about how information is documented on the patient's chart. Avoid use of slang terms and labels to describe the patient.

Slander

Slander is the injury of a person's character, name, or reputation by false and malicious spoken word. To avoid committing slander, limit reporting of patient information to only appropriate and authorized personnel.

Patient Consent

The American legal system guarantees that patients have the right to consent to or refuse the provision of medical care. When a patient registers in the ED, he or she will be asked to sign a general consent form for treatment. This type of consent has limitations. Often, if additional invasive procedures or surgery is required, an additional consent is necessary. Failure to obtain patient permission or consent may result in charges of battery against the health care worker, but emergency lifesaving treatments are never withheld due to lack of consent.

Informed Consent

This type of consent is obtained by explaining all of the risks, benefits, and alternatives to the specific treatment to the patient. Under the theory of informed consent, the patient or the patient's family must have everything explained. The nurse or physician provides the information, and the patient decides whether or not to undergo the procedure or treatment. The patient must have decision-making capability and understand exactly the care and treatment he or she is agreeing to receive. Appropriate informed consent includes discussion of the nature of the illness or injury, the recommended treatment and associated risks, alternative treatment and risks, and the danger of refusing treatment. Examples include consent for surgery, invasive procedures, medications, and alternative therapies. Most often informed consent must be documented, signed, and witnessed.

Implied Consent

This type of consent is not necessarily stated by the patient or obtained in written form. When a patient is unable to give permission for treatment due to injury, illness, or mental status, implied consent is permitted when withholding treatment may cause the patient harm. To put it another way, if the patient was able to give consent, he or she would choose to allow the ED staff to take the necessary steps to save his or her life. Conditions that may call for implied permission include unconsciousness, altered mental status from drugs, alcohol, trauma, shock, or mental illness.

Consents for Minors or Pediatric Patients

For patients who are younger than the state's legal age, consent may be obtained from the parent or legal guardian. Legal age may vary from state to state, and it is important to know what the age of majority is in your state. Some states also have special legislation that allows a minor to obtain medical treatment for specific conditions, such as pregnancy, psychiatric illness, drug, or alcohol treatment, and treatment of sexually transmitted diseases.

Additionally, some minors are considered emancipated. Emancipated minors can give permission for treatment. Criteria for being declared an emancipated minor include living independently of parents, being self-supporting or married, serving in the United States armed forces, or being pregnant. In many states, the patient must have a court decree to be declared an emancipated minor.

Involuntary Consent

This type of consent is supplied by process of the law. Typically it is used for prisoners or individuals under arrest who require medical examination or treatment. The scope of treatment is limited.

Right to Refuse Treatment

Patients have the right to refuse all or parts of their treatment at any time. To refuse, a patient must be determined to have decision-making capability to understand the situation and alternatives, be able to communicate a decision, and be able to understand the consequences of the decision.

Examples in which the patient may not have the decision-making capability to refuse treatment include mental impairment by alcohol, drugs, or mental illness.

Sometimes, a patient may wish to leave a hospital before treatment is completed or against medical advice (AMA). In cases of refusal or AMA, the ET should inform the nurse or physician, who then assess the situation and takes appropriate action. Decisions to detain or physically restrain a patient for treatment are made by the physician.

Documentation

Every patient who comes to the ED deserves a thorough and accurate medical record. Thorough documentation of the patient's signs, symptoms, and treatment may be the primary responsibility of the nurses and physicians. Some hospitals, however, may require the ET to document certain patient-related information such as vital signs. Therefore, the ET should understand a few simple principles associated with documentation. Information that should be documented in the medical record is listed below.

- Dates
- Times
- The patient's physical condition, including results of a primary and secondary survey
- The patient's medical history
- Any treatment administered in the ED
- Any reaction or lack of reaction from those treatments
- Any changes in vital signs or physical condition
- Any unusual circumstances or causes for delay in tests or treatments, such as the failure to obtain consent

- The mental status of the patient, with any changes, should be recorded on a regular basis, especially if the patient has sustained a head injury.

- All airway maintenance procedures, as well as use of any supplemental oxygen devices, should be accurately and consistently recorded.

- If the patient sustains any spinal or possible spinal cord injury, the movement and sensation of all the extremities must be recorded. Any changes must be documented.

- Any violent or unusual behaviors should be listed, with care to avoid using terms such as drunk or crazy.

Any information that is documented should be an objective account of patient observations. Most important, all handwriting should be legible. The ET may be required to testify to the care given or symptoms observed years after the event.

Some EDs make photographic records for certain patients. Photographs are often taken in cases of abuse, neglect, or suspected criminal cases. It is important that consent be obtained for the photographs, that the patient's privacy and dignity be protected, and that the photographs be attached to the proper medical records.

Confidentiality

All health care workers have the moral and legal obligation to maintain patient confidentiality. Many hospitals specify that violation of patient confidentiality is grounds for dismissal. Ensuring that the patient's identity and medical condition are kept confidential is related to the patient's right to privacy and is covered under invasion of privacy as well as slander and libel considerations. Civil suits may be brought against health care providers for the failure to maintain confidentiality. Share the patient information on a "need-to-know" basis only. That is, share information with other health care providers only as much as they need that information to take care of the patient. Do not publicly discuss sensitive and private information. Do not give information without the patient's permission.

Mandated Reporting

Most hospitals and health agencies are required by state law to report specific conditions to the state, law enforcement agencies, or health agencies. Examples include child or elder maltreatment; domestic violence; specific infectious diseases; animal bites; violent crimes, including gunshot wounds, stab wounds, and rape or criminal sexual assault; and successful or attempted suicide. Reporting these conditions is not the direct responsibility of the ET; however, any information obtained during the course of a conversation with a patient must be shared with the nurse or physician. While patient confidentiality must be preserved, the duty to report protects both the patient and the public.

Emergency Medical Treatment and Labor Act

The ET, who functions as an assistant to the registered nurse at triage, also must be aware of the federal Emergency Medical Treatment and Labor Act (EMTALA) legislation. Components of this law address intrafacility patient transfer, patient stabilization, and access to emergency care. The ET must recognize that under the EMTALA legislation, all patients who come to the ED for treatment must undergo a medical screening examination prior to transfer to another facility.

In addition, this examamination must take place before any information about the patient's ability or intent to pay for services is obtained. Failure to comply with the legislation may result in large fines for the institution and revocation of certain privileges and federal reimbursements.

Summary

Knowledge of legal issues helps the ET provide patient care that is both safe and legal. Undoubtedly, other issues of a legal nature may surface in the course of patient care. The recommended best practice or action for the ET is to adhere to his or her job description, specific institutional policies, and seek specific direction from the nurse or supervisor.

Bibliography

American College of Legal Medicine. (2001). *Legal medicine.* (5th ed.). St. Louis, MO: Mosby.

Brent, N. (2001). *Nurses and the law: A guide to principles and applications* (2nd ed.). Philadelphia: Saunders.

Emergency Nurses Association. (1998). *Emergency nursing pediatric course provider manual.* (2nd ed.). Park Ridge, IL: Author.

Emergency Nurses Association. (2000). *Emergency nursing core curriculum.* (5th ed.). Philadelphia: Saunders.

Goldstein, A. S. (1983). *EMS and the law: A legal handbook for EMS personnel.* Bowie, MD: Robert J. Brady Co.

Hall, J. K. (1996). *Nursing ethics and the law.* Philadelphia: Saunders.

McQuillan, K.A., Von Rueden, K.T., Hartsock, R.L., Flynn, M.B., and Whalen, E. (2002). *Trauma nursing from resuscitation through rehabilitation.* (3rd ed.). Philadelphia: Saunders.

Romano, J. (1998). *Legal rights of the catastrophically ill and injured: A family guide.* (2nd ed.). Norristown, PA: Author.

Objectives

Upon completion of this module, the learner should be able to:

- Describe safe patient lifting and moving techniques.
- State the principles of proper body mechanics.
- Identify four ways to prevent back injuries.

Chapter 15

Body Mechanics

Introduction

The Emergency Technician (ET) is expected to carry, move, and transport supplies and patients from various locations. The ability to safely move patients and supplies depends on the use of proper body mechanics. Health care providers become so focused on the patients in their care that sometimes they forget the importance of using proper body mechanics; failure to do so may cause serious injury.

Proper Posture and Body Mechanics

Posture directly affects the ligaments of the back, particularly those in the lower back. Slouching, over time, puts pressure on the vertebrae, which can eventually cause back strain. The best way to prevent strain is to use proper posture. This includes standing with the head up, shoulders back, chest out, stomach in, and buttocks tucked.

Back injury is the most common cause of work-related injuries. According to the United States Department of Labor, more than 1 million workers suffer a back injury every year. Three out of four of these injuries occur while lifting.

Patient Handling

Explain procedures before moving a patient. An unexplained, sudden movement may startle the patient, placing the patient and the ET at risk for injury. The ET must recognize his or her own physical abilities and limitations, and when necessary, ask for additional help. In addition, be aware of the resources available inside and outside of the ED. For example, a pull sheet or transfer board placed under a patient makes it easier to move him or her from bed to bed when limited help is available (see

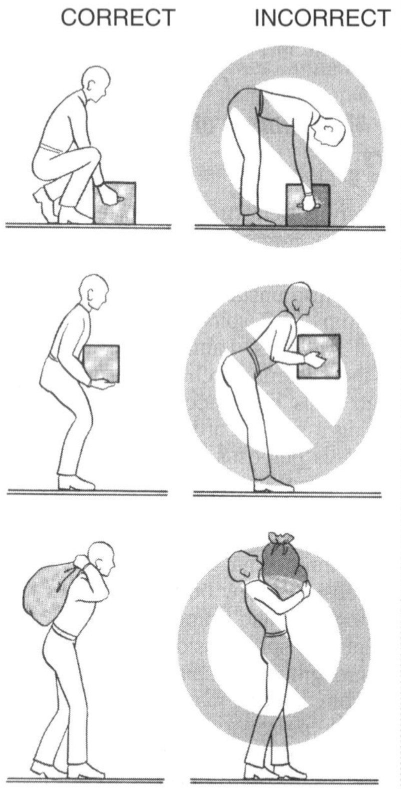
CORRECT
INCORRECT

Figure 15-1 Proper Body Mechanics

(Reprinted with permission from: Schnell, S. S. (1993). Nursing care of clients with disorders of the spinal cord, peripheral nerves, and cranial nerves. In Black, J. M., & Jacobs, E. M. (Eds.). *Luckmann and Sorensen's Medical-surgical nursing: A psychophysiologic approach* (4th ed., p. 815). Philadelphia: Saunders.)

Tips for good body mechanics (see **Figure 15-1**):

- Bend at the knees and hips, not at the waist, to pick up objects.
- Avoid lifting objects above shoulder level or below the waist.
- Push a load using your body's weight whenever possible; pulling can cause muscle strain.
- Never lift a load that is too heavy; get help.
- Pivot the whole body; do not twist at the waist.
- Keep objects close to the body. When lifting, tighten stomach muscles to protect the back. Let the legs do the work, not the back or arms.
- Do not overreach for an object; move closer to the object before picking it up.

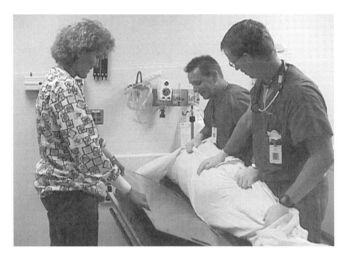

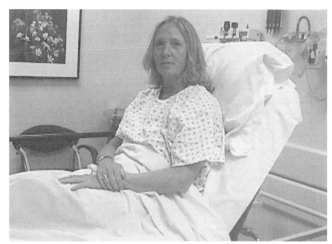

Figure 15-2 Slide Board and Proper Positioning Around Bed

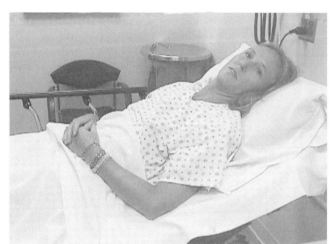

Figure 15-2). Additional transfer equipment, such as patient lifts, may be borrowed from other patient care areas.

The patient's airway is a very important factor to consider during any transport. A patient who is lying flat (supine) with a pillow under the head may look comfortable, but this may be the worst position for a patient with respiratory problems (see **Figure 15-3**). In most cases, a conscious patient with breathing problems is placed in an upright sitting position.

Review the following when positioning a patient:

Safety

- *Patient's level of consciousness:* Is the patient awake and alert or does he or she have an altered level of consciousness?

- *Side rails:* Are they locked in the upright position?

- *Call bell:* Is it within the patient's reach?

- *Seizure precautions:* Is there a need for special rail padding?

- *Suction:* Is suction readily available and functioning?

- *Oxygen:* Does the patient require oxygen?

- *Other tubes and wires:* Does the patient have IVs or other tubes (i.e., catheters, chest tube, pulse oximetry, telemetry leads) connected to the body that may be affected during a position change?

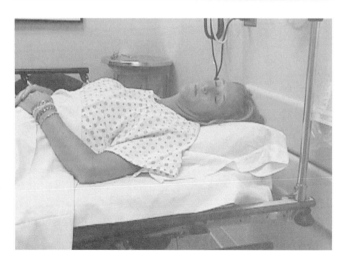

Figure 15-3 High Fowler's, SemiFowler's and Supine

- *Areas of injury:* Is the patient injured? Avoid placing the patient on the affected area of injury, as this may cause additional pain as well as further damage to that area.

- *Areas of immobilization:* Are there areas that require immobilization? If so, maintain immobilization during positioning to prevent further musculoskeletal and/or neurologic damage.

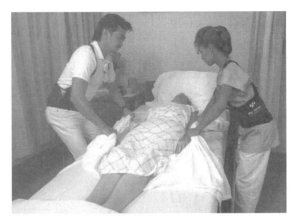

A. Moving patient up in bed.

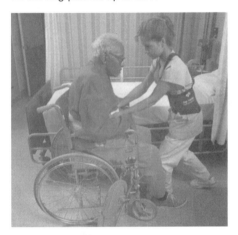

B. Moving patient from wheelchair to bed.

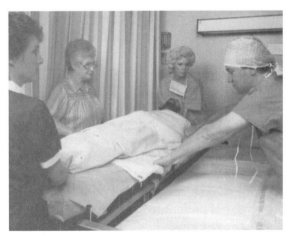

C. Moving patient from stretcher to bed.

Figure 15-4 A, B, C Types of Transfers.

(Reprinted with permission from: Hegner, B., & Caldwell, E. (1995). Body mechanics. In *Nursing assistant: A nursing process approach* (7th ed., p. 207, 213, 218). Albany, NY: Delmar Publishers.)

Patient Communication

- Does the patient understand how or why to use the call bell?
- Explain why the patient must not get up.
- Explain the reason for the position change.

Team Communication

- Discuss with the nurse or physician any patient positioning concerns.
- Assist the team with evaluating how the patient tolerates the position.
- Notify the nurse of any change in the patient's condition.
- Identify how often a position change is required (such as for the patient who is restrained).

Extremity Positions

- Elevate an injured arm or leg by placing one or two pillows beneath the limb, unless directed otherwise by the nurse or physician.
- Immobilize the extremity to prevent further movement under the direction of the nurse.

Patient Transfers

- Is more than one person needed to accomplish this?
- Is the patient cooperative?
- Are there any tubes, wires, or other equipment that requires the nurse be present for the transfer?
- Are there any body parts that need to be immobilized before transfer?
- Is there additional equipment that must be brought with the patient during the transfer (i.e., cardiac monitor, portable suction, IV poles)?
- Which mode of transportation will be best suited for this particular transfer (i.e., stretcher, wheelchair)?

Types of transfers (see **Figure 15-4**):
- Wheelchair to stretcher
- Stretcher or wheelchair to hospital bed
- Wheelchair to vehicle
- Stretcher to wheelchair
- Stretcher to stretcher
- Vehicle to wheelchair or stretcher
- Moving patient up in bed or stretcher, logrolling onto or off a backboard

Material Handling

The ET is expected to stock and move supplies. Some supplies, such as gauze pads, are lightweight, whereas some items, such as a carton of crutches, weigh much more. Many people have been misled to believe that the weight of the object lifted or moved determines the risk for injury. This is a myth, and it is important to understand why. A person can lift cartons that weigh 50 pounds every day for years without apparent injury. Then one day, while bending over to pick up the soap in the shower, he or she cannot stand up without back pain. Was it the soap that caused the injury? No, it was the cumulative effect of many years of repeated use of incorrect body mechanics to pick things up or move objects that weakened the back and set the stage for injury. Therefore, it is extremely important to use proper body mechanics.

Summary

All members of the ED health care team are at risk for back injuries if they use improper body mechanics. The ET is especially at risk for this type of injury due to the nature of the job specifications. Planning actions and recognizing situations that require help from another person or a tool is the best defense against injury.

Bibliography

Agsafe, The Safety Center. (1997). Body mechanics and patient transfers. *Back Injury Prevention.* Berkley, CA: Author. (www.usbm.gov/niosh/nasd/docs/as32900.html)

Shade, B., Rothenburg, M.A., Wertz, E., & Jones, S. (1997). *Mosby's EMT intermediate textbook.* St. Louis, MO: Mosby-Year Book.

US Department of Labor. (1997). *Back injuries—Nation's #1 workplace safety problem.* Springfield, Virginia: The National Technical Information Service. www.pp.okstate.edu/ehs/training/oshaback.html.

Chapter 16

Infection Control and Personal Protection

Introduction

All members of the health care team are at risk for exposure to infectious diseases. The most powerful prevention tool is knowledge. Knowledge, combined with strict infection control precautions, provides the greatest protection against exposure.

Microorganisms

Microorganisms are so small they can be seen only with a microscope. Some microorganisms found in the human body are beneficial. Others, however, can produce disease and infection. Microorganisms can originate in many places of the body, such as the skin or mucous membranes. Others may come from an outside source such as the environment. Examples of various types of organisms are listed below:

- Bacteria

- Viruses

- Fungi

- Protozoa

Modes of Transmission

Microorganisms that cause infection are spread in four principal ways:

- Droplet or Airborne: Sneezing, coughing, and even talking can send microscopic droplets through the air. Diseases that can spread through droplet transmission include the following:
  - Chickenpox
  - Measles
  - Mumps
  - Tuberculosis
  - Influenza
  - Some types of pneumonia
  - Common cold

Covering the mouth or nose when sneezing or coughing helps prevent the transmission of airborne droplets. Patients with a disease that is spread by droplet transmission should have a mask placed over their mouth and nose to prevent additional transmission. This precaution will protect patients in adjacent treatment areas and health care providers working in close proximity to the infected patient.

- Direct Contact: Touching secretions, clothing, bedding, or a dressing can result in the transmission of an infection. The Emergency Technician (ET) should anticipate the potential for contact with infected fluids when caring for patients and take the appropriate safety measures. The following bodily fluids should always be considered infectious.
  - Blood
  - Urine
  - Stool
  - Sputum
  - Vaginal and penile secretions
  - Cerebrospinal fluid
  - Synovial fluid
  - Pleural fluid
  - Peritoneal fluid
  - Amniotic fluid

- Ingestion: Anything that is ingested, such as water, food, or foreign objects, may carry microorganisms that produce illness or an infectious disease.

- Animals or Insects: Infectious microorganisms can be transmitted to humans from animals or insects. Lyme disease (deer tick) and malaria (mosquito) are commonly recognized diseases transmitted via insects. Infections transmitted through animals have dramatically decreased; however, rabies remains the most notable example.

Defense Mechanisms

The skin plays an important role in preventing microorganisms from invading the body. Areas in which the skin is no longer intact, such as scrapes or open wounds, become an entry point for microorganisms, which can then result in infection.

The ability of the body to fight infection is directly related to the general health and immune system of the individual. If a person's health is poor or the immune system is compromised (i.e., a cancer patient on chemotherapy), the chance of successfully fighting an infection is markedly reduced.

Asepsis and Sterile Technique

Asepsis is the absence of microorganisms. Surgical asepsis (sterile technique) is a procedure that eliminates *all* organisms, both good and bad, from objects or areas. Sterilization of supplies and equipment destroys *all* microorganisms by heat, chemicals, or gases. Sterile technique should be used whenever a patient is at risk for exposure, such as by a break in the skin or an invasive procedure. Situations that necessitate the use of sterile technique include suturing wounds, burn care, or inserting a urinary catheter.

Medical asepsis or "clean technique" is a procedure that cleans the object or area but does not destroy all the microorganisms. Use of antimicrobial agents, such as soaps and detergents, that kill or slow the growth of harmful microorganisms is an example.

Handwashing is another form of medical asepsis and considered the single most effective way to prevent the spread of infection. The following steps are required for effective handwashing.

- Wet hands with warm water.
- Apply soap and rub the fingers, the back and front of the hands, and between the fingers. Rub the hands together for one minute. The friction is essential in removing microorganisms.
- Rinse the hands thoroughly with warm water.
- Dry the hands thoroughly with a paper towel.
- Use a paper towel to turn off the faucet.

To ensure that infection is not spread, handwashing is performed at specific times, as listed below.

- On arrival to work and on departure
- Before and after every contact with every patient
- After any contact with blood or bodily fluids
- Before and after eating
- After using the bathroom
- After removing protective gloves
- After putting hands to the face to cough, sneeze, or blow the nose

Jewelry must not be worn during working hours. Microorganisms easily become trapped underneath rings. Rings and bracelets can pierce the examination or procedure gloves. A microscopic hole in a glove will allow potentially infectious fluids to pass through.

Bodily Fluids

Protective equipment must be worn in all situations where there is the possibility of coming in contact with potentially contaminated bodily fluids. The following bodily fluids can contain microorganisms that are easily spread if protective equipment is not worn.

- Blood
- Feces
- Urine
- Sweat
- Sputum
- Tears
- Vomitus
- Saliva
- Nasal secretions
- Semen

Personal Protective Equipment (PPE)

Disposable Gloves

Sterile and nonsterile gloves are available in different sizes. Sterile (or surgical) gloves are used for procedures such as suturing, performing a lumbar puncture, or any other sterile field procedure. Although the physician does these procedures, the ET may be asked to assist. Always ask if sterile gloves are needed. Nonsterile (or examination) gloves are used when touching a patient's skin or coming into contact with bodily fluids, as well as when transporting or handling specimens. These gloves are worn one time only and most commonly come in vinyl and latex. These gloves must be changed when soiled and after every patient contact. The same pair of gloves must never be used for contact between two patients.

The ET should be aware of any personal sensitivity or allergy to latex and inform the nurse or supervisor about it immediately. Avoid hand lotions that are oil-based when wearing latex gloves. The oil in the lotion breaks down the latex, decreasing the glove's ability to provide barrier protection. Remember that the purpose of glove wearing is to protect you from an exposure to an infectious agent. Should a glove tear or become punctured while in use, and you are exposed to a potential harmful agent, follow the institution's exposure policy.

Remember to remove gloves in the following order: Dirty to dirty and clean to clean (see **Figure 16-1**). Bare hands are considered clean so they should only touch clean surfaces inside the glove. By removing gloves inside out, contaminated surfaces stay together. Dispose of the gloves in the hazardous waste garbage receptacle, which is easily identified by the bright red plastic biohazard bag.

Disposable Masks

Masks are used as a barrier to droplet microorganisms. Depending on the situation, either the health care provider or the patient may wear a mask. A patient who has an uncontrollable cough from a potentially infectious agent such as tuberculosis may wear a mask. The health care provider may wear a mask to maintain a sterile area.

Figure 16-1 Removing Dirty Gloves

Reprinted with permission from: Hegner, B., & Caldwell, E. (1995). Basic media asepsis. In *Nursing assistant: A nursing process approach* (7th ed., p. 161). Albany, NY: Delmar Publishers.

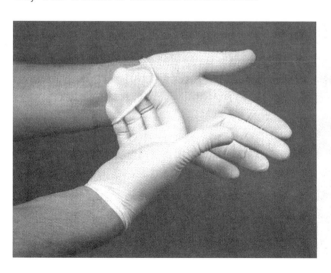
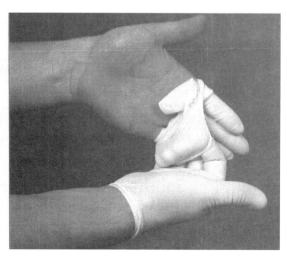

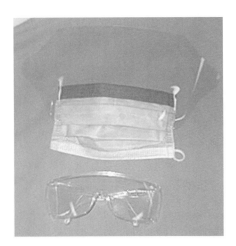

Figure 16-2 Goggles and Splash Shields

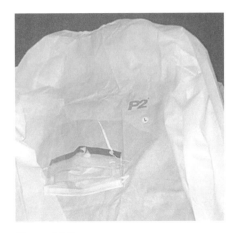

Figure 16-3 Gown

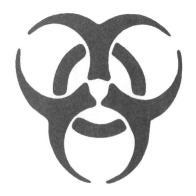

Figure 16-4 Biohazard Symbol

There are various types of masks. Become familiar with the types of masks used in your hospital and learn the situations appropriate for each type. A personal protective mask may be fitted and used as a tuberculosis barrier.

Eye Protection

The mucous membranes of the eyes (conjunctiva) can be easily splashed with blood and bodily fluids. Wearing goggles with side protectors will help prevent this from happening (see **Figure 16-2**). Ordinary prescription glasses do not offer enough protection unless they have side protectors. Keep a pair of protective goggles and/or splash shield available at all times.

Disposable Gowns

Disposable gowns are worn over the uniform or scrubs to provide protection from exposure to blood or body fluids (see **Figure 16-3**). Gowns should be used when caring for trauma patients or patients with any type of exposed bodily fluid or secretions.

Supplies, such as gloves, masks, gowns, and eye protection, must be readily accessible to health care team members at all times. Follow your hospital's policy that identifies when to use them.

The Occupational Safety and Health Administration (OSHA) has rules for workplace safety that health care facilities are required to follow. These rules not only include the protective devices discussed in this chapter, but they also refer to a standard of practice when caring for patients. This standard involves either universal or standard precautions. These standards will be reviewed during orientation.

The wording of the standards may vary from one hospital to another; however, the intent is the same. Every patient must be approached as a potential carrier of an infectious disease. The role of the ET is to be aware of this potential and to make no assumptions about which patients may or may not be carriers. Infectious diseases, such as hepatitis and human immunodeficiency virus (HIV), do not discriminate on the basis of gender, race, or age.

Disposal Containers

Hospitals have policies on where and how to dispose of contaminated materials. Patient clothing that has been contaminated with blood or other bodily fluids should be separated from the other laundry. Dressings, tubing, and other supplies with blood or bodily fluids should be disposed of in trash containers with red liners showing the biohazard symbol (see **Figure 16-4**). Every hospital has established policies governing disposal. It is the ET's responsibility to become familiar with the specific policies and procedures of his or her hospital.

Another disposal concern is that of sharp objects, such as needles, IV catheters, and suturing materials. Be very alert and cautious when preparing the patient care area. Needles are easily hidden under a sponge or towel. Always wear gloves and dispose of sharp items in a container specifically designed for these items.

The following guidelines assist in maintaining safe work practices.

- Never recap a needle.

- Do not eat or drink in work areas.

- Do not handle personal items such as contact lenses in the work area.
- Clean up all blood or bodily fluid spills promptly.
- Always wear gloves when the potential for an exposure exists.
- Use plastic bags to transport specimens.
- Be aware of the policies and procedures in the ED that relate to blood and bodily fluids.
- Be aware of the appropriate chemical used to clean equipment and spills.
- Do not wear uniforms outside the work area. Leave work shoes at the hospital as well.
- Use personal protective devices (gloves, masks, gowns).
- Develop a good handwashing routine.
- Use a barrier device for mouth-to-mouth cardiopulmonary resuscitation (CPR).

Personal Hygiene

Just as the ET must be protected from a patient who may be the source of an infection, the patient also must be protected from the health care worker with a potential infection. An ET who has cuts or abrasions on the hands must report it to the nurse or supervisor and wear gloves as directed. The hospital may have policies regarding limitations on reporting to work with strep throat, conjunctivitis, and other illnesses. Any draining wounds must be covered completely and reported to the supervisor of employee health.

Summary

The spread of infectious organisms can cause illness to the ET or patients. Understanding how transmission occurs and following institutional, as well as OSHA guidelines, will help prevent infectious exposures. Proper handwashing technique is the single most effective way to ensure that contamination does not spread from patient to patient.

Bibliography

Ansell Medical. (1996). *Donning Techniques-Sterile Gloves.* www.ansellhealthcare.com/latex_gloves/what_you_should_know/E/ donning_techniques.html

Borton, D. (1997). Isolation precautions. *Nursing 97,* January, 49–51.

Shade, B., Rothenburg, M.A., Wertz, E., Jones, S. and Collins, T. (2002). *Mosby's EMT intermediate textbook.* St. Louis, MO: Mosby.

Upon completion of this module, the learner should be able to:

- Define phlebotomy.

- Select an appropriate site for venipuncture.

- Describe proper venipuncture techniques.

- Identify which collection tubes are used for each test and the contents of each tube.

- Describe proper skin puncture techniques and care of the site after the procedure is completed.

- Discuss proper specimen care.

Chapter 17

Phlebotomy

Introduction

Phlebotomy is a puncture made in the wall of a vein (venipuncture) to remove blood for testing. Selecting the proper site for venipuncture is essential to obtain a good specimen. Proper site selection will also decrease patient discomfort and complications. Even when phlebotomy is done correctly, possible hazards exist. Therefore, it is important for the Emergency Technician (ET) to recognize the possible hazards and be able to appropriately handle the situation. This section describes how the ET may safely and effectively obtain a blood specimen from patients in the emergency department (ED). The basic equipment required for obtaining and holding blood specimens are reviewed, although brand names of equipment vary among institutions.

Anatomy and Physiology of Blood

Blood is the fluid present in arteries and veins and accounts for about 8% of the body's mass. It is responsible for circulating nutrients, oxygen, hormones, and waste products throughout the body. Blood contains liquid and solid components.

Plasma

The liquid part of blood is known as plasma, which accounts for 55% of the blood volume. Plasma is primarily composed of water (91.5%), proteins (7%) such as albumins, globulins, and fibrinogen, and other solutes (1.5%) such as electrolytes, lipids, enzymes, clotting factors, and glucose.

Red Blood Cells

Red blood cells (erythrocytes), white blood cells, and platelets make up the other 45% of the blood's volume. Red blood cells are produced in the bone marrow and contain hemoglobin, a protein that binds with oxygen in the lungs and transports it to the body tissues.

White Blood Cells

White blood cells (leukocytes) function as part of the body's immune system. There are several different types of leukocytes, each with a separate function. However, all leukocytes share the common task of defending the body against foreign microorganisms and substances.

Platelets

Platelets help the blood to clot, which seals off ruptured blood vessels. When a blood vessel is injured, platelets are glued together with the protein fibrin to close off the ruptured vessel. A blood clot contains blood cells and clotting proteins. Serum is the liquid portion of a blood sample after a clot has formed.

Venipuncture

If a tray is used to hold all the necessary equipment for a venipuncture, make sure it is kept neat, well stocked, and disinfected periodically with a 10% bleach solution. The following equipment must be readily available to perform a venipuncture (see also **Figure 17-1**).

- Adhesive bandages
- Alcohol pads (sterile)
- Betadine pads (sterile)
- Blood collection tubes (small and large sizes)
- Capillary tubes
- Exam gloves
- Gauze sponges (2 × 2)
- Ink marking pen
- Lancets (sterile, for skin punctures)
- Needles (sterile)
- Sharps container
- Syringes (sterile) 3 and 5 ml
- Tourniquets—do not use latex tourniquets for patients who are latex sensitive
- Surgical tape

Blood Collection Tubes

Blood collection tubes are either plastic or glass and have colored stoppers. The colors are used to indicate the types of additive, if any, contained in the tube (see **Table 17-1**). Additives are necessary to perform different tests on the blood specimen. Tube additives either help initiate blood clotting (clot activators) or prevent blood clotting (anticoagulants). Clot activators are made of silica gel. Anticoagulants are either liquids or dry substances.

Gently mix any tube with an additive immediately after filling it with blood. This prevents the blood from clotting or ensures

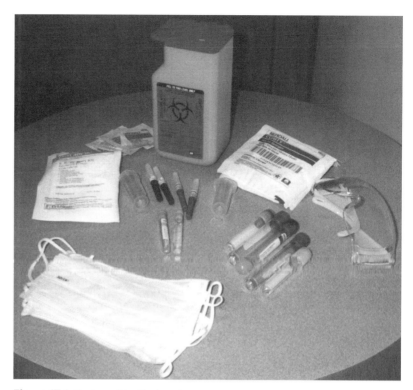

Figure 17-1 Equipment for Venipuncture
(Photographed by Donna Massey, RN, MSN.)

Table 17-1 Tube Tope Colors and Their Uses

Color	Type of Test
Red	Chemistry, immunology, and blood banking tests
Gold and red marbled	Chemistry tests
Light and dark green marbled	Chemistry tests
Lavender	Hematology tests
Light blue	Coagulation (clotting) studies
Dark blue	Trace elements, nutrients, or toxicology studies
Brown	Lead levels
Green	Viable lymphocytes or neutrophils Chemistry tests
Gray	Blood glucose or alcohol levels
Yellow	Pediatric blood cultures Blood bank, viable cells
Orange or yellow and gray marbled	Emergency (STAT) chemistry tests

Figure 17-2 Sample I.D. bands

(Reprinted with permission from: College of American Pathologists. (1999). Approaching the patient. In *So you're going to collect a blood specimen: An introduction to phlebotomy.* (8th ed., p. 14). Northfield, IL. Author.)

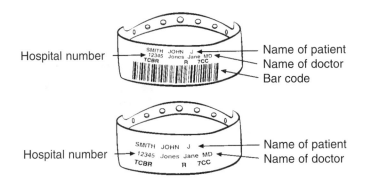

the proper distribution of a clot activator. The amount of additive is specific for the volume of blood in the tube. Tubes are vacuum sealed, or evacuated, and normally draw in the correct amount of blood. Overfilling or underfilling the tubes may affect test results.

When a tube is filled, invert it at least 10 times to mix anticoagulants and 5 times to distribute clot activator. Do not shake the tubes as blood cells may rupture, giving incorrect test results.

Patient and Test Identification

Prior to obtaining a blood specimen, all tubes and any other equipment needed to perform all requested tests should be sealed. When approaching a patient to obtain a blood specimen, the ET should introduce himself or herself to the correct patient. Ask the patient to state his or her name and verify the name on the patient's identification bracelet (see **Figure 17-2**). Do not rely on the patient's room number or bed number. The patient may have moved or the location mistakenly documented. Explain the procedure to the patient and provide reassurance. Sometimes patients are nervous about the amount of blood being drawn, especially if several tubes are needed.

Collection tubes should be labelled prior to drawing blood, as a tube labeled with a different patient's information may be used by mistake. After tubes are filled with blood, ensure that the tubes are labeled with the correct patient's information. This must be done in the patient's presence, if possible, to avoid questions about whether the specimens were labeled correctly.

Information required on tube labels and test requisition forms may vary by institutions. At a minimum, the patient's full name, date, and time of collection and the ET's initials should be included. If specimens are processed at another location, indicate the facility's identification information on the label and type of test required.

Selecting a Venipuncture Site

Venipuncture refers to collecting blood from a vein, not an artery. The veins in the arm typically are the first choice for blood collection because they are usually the easiest to find and to position; however, if these veins are inaccessible or undesirable, others may be used, such as those in the hands, wrists, or feet. Some institutions may require a physician's order to draw blood from the feet.

The arm veins most commonly used are located in the cubital fossa region (anterior bend of the elbow) of the arm (see **Figure 17-3**). These veins are the cephalic vein (laterally), basilic vein (medial), and the median vein (inferior to the basilic vein).

When selecting a vein to collect blood from, avoid thrombosed veins as these veins have clots and scar tissue inside, which makes collecting a specimen difficult. Thrombosed veins may have been damaged from repeated venipuncture or fluid injection. Thrombosed veins feel harder than normal veins and may cause the patient discomfort when touched.

Avoid collecting blood from a vein with a running IV, as the fluid may alter test results. If there is no choice but to collect blood from an arm with an IV, the specimen collection site must be below the IV site. Avoid collecting blood if cellulitis (inflammation of the skin) is present or from arm veins on the same side a mastectomy (breast removal) or a lumpectomy has been performed.

Hazards and Complications in Phlebotomy

Personal Safety

When collecting blood specimens, personal safety and the safety of the patient and coworkers are paramount. Practicing universal precautions at all times is critical to avoid exposure to bloodborne pathogens such as human immunodeficiency virus (HIV), hepatitis B, and others. Clean and disinfect any blood spills immediately. Wash hands with soap and water before and after each patient contact. Remove gloves after contact with each patient, and apply a new pair before working with a new patient.

If a contaminated needle pierces the skin, remove the gloves immediately. Squeeze the site to promote bleeding, which helps remove any contamination. Wash the site vigorously with soap and water. If blood splashes into the eyes, mucous membranes, or any open wounds, immediately flush the affected area with water. Document the patient's name and identification number on an incident report form. Inform the nurse of the exposure and follow the institution's policy on reporting and treatment.

Patient Safety

A hematoma is swelling that occurs as a result of bleeding beneath the skin. If a hematoma appears while collecting a blood specimen, stop the procedure immediately and apply pressure to the site with a cotton ball or gauze sponge for 5 minutes or until bleeding stops.

Hemolysis is the destruction of red blood cells, which may alter certain test results. To avoid hemolysis, allow the venipuncture site to dry after cleaning, do not use needles that are too small for blood collection, or draw from a hematoma. Mix tubes gently if additives are present so that blood cells are not damaged.

Some patients may become dizzy or experience syncope (fainting) during the procedure. The patient always must be seated in a chair or lying on a bed when blood is being drawn. The ET should be positioned in front of seated patients to prevent them from falling out of the chair if they faint. Watch patients closely after drawing blood, especially if they stand up. Patients who feel dizzy or light-headed should sit or lie down until they feel that they have recovered. Check with the nurse before offering the patient orange juice or water. Patients must not have anything in their mouth while having blood drawn as they may choke or aspirate if they faint.

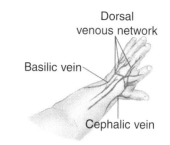

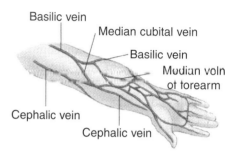

Figure 17-3 Veins in the Arm and Hand

(Reprinted with permission from: American Academy of Pediatrics. (2000). Intravenous access. In *Pediatric education for prehospital professionals* (p. 276). Elk Grove Village, IL: Author.)

Performing the Venipuncture

The patient must be sitting or lying down for easy access to the venipuncture site with a pillow or another object under the arm to help position and stabilize it. Veins sometimes appear bluish and may protrude slightly above the skin surface; however, it is not necessary to see the vein to access the site. Many veins are easily palpated without being visible.

To find a suitable vein, apply a tourniquet to the upper arm, half way between the shoulder and elbow. The tourniquet must be tight enough to stop venous blood flow but not impede arterial flow. Ask the patient to open and close a fist to fill the veins with blood. Veins feel like spongy, elastic tubes. If there is a pulse, the vessel is an artery, not a vein. Thrombosed veins feel rigid and, as discussed earlier, must be avoided. Check both arms before deciding on a vein. The patient may be able to identify a good site, especially if blood has been drawn in the past. If you have trouble finding a vein, use a pen light to locate the veins, especially in infants and children. A warm, moist cloth wrapped around the arm also may increase blood flow and make the veins easier to see and feel.

Before obtaining a blood specimen, attach a new, sterile needle to the needle holder and gather the necessary evacuated tubes. Inspect the needle for burrs or nicks and discard if necessary. If using a syringe or Butterfly™ IV needle, carefully transfer the blood into evacuated tubes after completing the draw. When searching for a vein, do not leave the tourniquet in place for more than two minutes. When collecting a specimen, the tourniquet must not be tied for more than four to five minutes, or the test results may be altered.

After a good vein is located, use a new alcohol pad or betadine pad to wipe the site in an outward circular motion. Allow the area to air dry or wipe it with gauze. Do not blow on the site, as this recontaminates it.

To keep the vein from moving, use the thumb or index finger to pull the skin tight on the side of the vein or just below the draw site. Keep the needle parallel to the vein, at a 15-degree angle, with the bevel (flattened area at the tip of the needle) facing up (see **Figure 17-4**).

Puncture the vein with a smooth motion. Once the needle is inside the vein, lower the angle of the needle and then advance the needle slightly into the vein. Keep the needle holder firmly in place and push an evacuated tube into it until the inner needle punctures the cap and the tube fills with blood. Remove the tube when it is full, but keep the needle in place until all necessary tubes have been filled.

Be sure to mix all tubes containing additives. With practice, this can be done while the next tube is filling. If the tourniquet has been on approxi-

Figure 17-4 Needle with Bevel Up to Draw From Site

(Reprinted with permission from: College of American Pathologists. (1996). The venipuncture from an arm vein. In *So you're going to collect a blood specimen: An introduction to phlebotomy* (8th ed., p. 20). Northfield, IL: Author.)

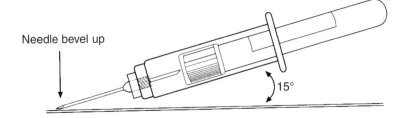

Needle bevel up

15°

mately four to five minutes, release it and continue collecting blood. After the last tube has been removed, remove the tourniquet, then the needle, and place a gauze pad on the site. Apply pressure until bleeding stops. Instruct the patient not to bend the arm because this may increase bleeding under the skin and cause bruising. When the bleeding stops, apply an adhesive bandage. Some patients may bleed excessively because of a medical condition or medications. For patients with excessive bleeding, apply pressure for more than five minutes. Elevating the arm also helps stop the bleeding. When bleeding has stopped, apply a small pressure dressing by folding the gauze pad and applying tape over the site. Do not wrap tape completely around the arm because this may cut off circulation.

Dispose of the needle and any wasted tubes into a puncture-resistant sharps container, also known as a biohazard container. Do not recap the needle. Label all the filled collection tubes before leaving the patient.

When drawing multiple samples, fill the tubes in the following order to reduce specimen contamination:

- Blood culture tubes
- Tubes without additives
- Coagulation tube (light blue stopper)
- Serum separator or clot activator tube
- Thrombin tube
- Heparin tube
- Gray top tube (blood glucose and alcohol levels)

Troublehsooting

Puncture Through the Vein

If blood fails to enter the tube, make sure that the needle has advanced into the vein but not too far to puncture the other side of the vein. Slowly withdraw the needle to see if blood appears in the tube. Palpate the position of the needle in relation to the vein and adjust the angle or direction of the needle insertion. If the vein has not been punctured, release the tourniquet, disconnect the tube from the Vacutainer™ or needle holder, and then remove the needle from the site. Identify another vein and attempt the venipuncture with a new needle and tube. If still unable to draw blood, stop the procedure and inform the nurse.

Arterial Puncture

Bright red blood pulsating into the tube is from an artery, not a vein. Arterial blood does not give the same test results as venous blood. Release the tourniquet and withdraw the needle. Apply pressure with a gauze pad until the bleeding has stopped and discard the needle and collected blood in a sharps or biohazard container.

Difficult Access

Elderly and pediatric patients typically have small or fragile veins. There also may be problems drawing blood from patients who have had chemotherapy or those with sickle cell disease because their veins have been damaged from repeated venipunctures. If this should happen, consider using a Butterfly™ IV needle or a needle and syringe instead of an evacuated tube. These devices allow more control of needle insertion and the amount of vacuum pressure applied on a vein. If using a needle and syringe to obtain blood from a child, make sure the syringe is no larger than 3 ml; anything larger may affect hemolysis or distort test results.

If unable to obtain a blood sample or access a vein successfully after two attempts, notify the nurse. Continued unsuccessful attempts only increase patient anxiety and discomfort.

Special Access Sites

Intravascular catheters are flexible tubes that are inserted into a patient's vein or artery. When collecting blood from these catheters, care must be taken to avoid causing an infection or hemorrhage (bleeding). Do not collect blood from these devices unless the ET has been specifically trained to do so.

A fistula is an artery connected to a vein. A vascular graft is a transplanted vein. Only specially trained personnel may use these sites. If blood must be collected from a vein with IV fluids entering it, perform the venipuncture below the infusion site. Document the type of fluid infusing.

Heel Puncture

When performing a heel puncture on infants (9 kg or 18 lbs or less), avoid touching the bone with the lancet, as this can cause inflammation and permanent disability. A warm towel wrapped around the foot may be used to increase circulation in the heel.

Special Tests

Blood culture tubes are used to test the amount of bacteria present in a patient's blood. Thoroughly clean the skin before drawing blood to prevent bacteria on the skin from interfering with test results. Follow the same procedures previously outlined for performing a venipuncture, and after thoroughly cleansing the puncture site with an alcohol wipe, cleanse it again with a betadine pad. Be sure not to touch the site after cleaning it. If a patient is sensitive to iodine, clean the site with an alcohol wipe for 10 seconds, let dry, and then clean with another alcohol wipe for another 10 seconds. Remember to label the tubes after filling them with blood.

The ET also may be involved in assisting with collecting specimens for blood alcohol testing for legal purposes, as in a car crash that resulted in a death. The police officer will have a special tube for collecting this type of specimen. Clean the site with a betadine pad; never use an alcohol wipe as the alcohol on the pad may interfere with the results.

Skin Punctures

Blood may be obtained by puncturing the skin rather than a vein. Some tests, such as blood glucose levels, may be done with capillary blood from a skin puncture. A skin puncture may also be used for patients whose veins are damaged, covered, or inaccessible. The middle and ring fingers are the preferred sites for skin puncture in adults. In infants, the heel is preferred. Avoid sites with scars, calluses, or lesions as blood is difficult to obtain from these areas; drawing from lesions may introduce an infection.

Grasp the desired finger with the thumb and index finger and with the opposite hand, gently massage toward the tip of the finger. Clean the fingertip with an alcohol wipe. Hold the finger, with the lancet on the outer anterior portion of the finger and puncture the skin with one smooth motion, making sure the cut is made perpendicular to the fingerprints. Dispose of the used lancet in a puncture-resistant sharps container.

Wipe away the first drop of blood with sterile gauze pad to avoid contamination in the specimen. Hold the finger down and apply gentle pressure to increase blood flow. To collect blood in micro collection tubes, simply allow blood to run into the tube. Cap the tube when full. If collecting blood into capillary tubes, place the open end of the tube horizontally into the drop of blood as it flows into the tube. Fill the tube $2/3$ to $3/4$ full. Cap the tube when full. If collecting blood onto a slide or a glucose testing strip, let a drop fall onto the desired location.

When using collection tubes, first collect the hematology specimen, then the chemistry specimen, then blood bank specimens. Collection in this order minimizes platelet clumping. Label the specimens on the container. Be sure to document that the samples are from a skin puncture.

Timed Specimens

The physician may order a single blood specimen to be collected from a patient at a specific time of day. Single or multiple collections also may be drawn at several different specific times throughout a given day or days. Several reasons exist for obtaining timed specimens. The accuracy of test results depends on collecting the blood at the exact specified time. Blood tests may be requested for patients with diabetes after they have eaten a meal. These requests may be documented "post cibum" (pc) or "post prandial" (pp). Blood glucose levels also may be checked at certain times to measure the effects of insulin treatments. Drug levels may be checked to measure the effects. After collecting a timed specimen, document the exact time the specimen is obtained.

Summary

Phlebotomy has potential risks and complications for the patient and the ET. Therefore, attention to detail and technique is important to perform phlebotomy without exposure to bloodborne pathogens or complications. Understanding how to effectively and safely collect blood samples from patients will decease patient discomfort and minimize the time a patient needs to spend in the ED.

Bibliography

Carter, P., & Pollakoff, J. (1996). *Phlebotomy skills manual.* Unpublished. UCLA Center For Prehospital Care.

College of American Pathologists. (1996). *So you're going to collect a blood specimen: An introduction to phlebotomy.* Northfield, IL: Author.

Lammon, C., Foote, A., Leli, P., Ingle, J., & Adams, M. (1995). *Clinical nursing skills.* Philadelphia: Saunders.

Pollakoff, J. (1996). *Blood withdrawal: Performance objectives.* Unpublished. UCLA Center For Prehospital Care.

Raven, P., & Johnson, G. (1995). *Biology* (3rd ed.). Dubuque, IA: Brown Publishers.

Tortora, G., Grabowski, S.R. (2000). *Introduction to the human body: The essentials of anatomy and physiology* (5th ed.) New York: John Wiley & Sons, Inc.

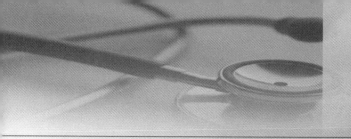

Hazardous Materials

Upon completion of this module, the learner should be able to:

- Describe the role of the Emergency Technician (ET) in the care of patients who are exposed to hazardous materials (HAZMAT).

- Identify the dangers to caregivers and the necessary precautions to care for patients exposed to hazardous materials.

- Identify three signs and symptoms that indicate a patient has been exposed to hazardous materials.

Introduction

A hazardous material is any substance that has the potential to cause harm to people or property. Hazardous materials may be chemical, radioactive, or even biological. Exposure to hazardous materials can result in a wide range of effects, from minor skin irritation to cardiorespiratory compromise and even death. Certain hazardous materials, such as asbestos, cause chronic illnesses, such as chronic obstructive pulmonary disease (COPD). Some agents cause changes in gene structure, which may lead to birth defects.

Even the smallest emergency department (ED) may receive patients who have been exposed to hazardous materials. Large quantities of hazardous materials are transported daily on US highways. Many hazardous materials are used in industry as well as in the home. Common household items, such as paint thinner, mercury thermometers, fertilizers and pesticides, bleach, toilet bowl cleaners, and batteries, are potentially harmful if ingested, inhaled, or absorbed through the skin.

In an effort to help patients, emergency personnel do not always consider the risks to their own health. Thus, the ED should have an action plan for patients exposed to hazardous material, and staff who are well educated in their roles and responsibilities related to HAZMAT. Hospitals need to be aware of the chemicals used in the industries in their area, develop care plans, and identify antidotes, if available, for the specific contaminants.

Often prehospital personnel initiate the decontamination process; however, patients may come to the ED by private vehicle instead of by ambulance. In some instances emergency medical services (EMS) personnel may transport a severely ill or injured patient to the ED without having had the time or the ability to decontaminate.

Identification of Hazardous Materials

There are numerous resources available to identify hazardous materials and their toxic effects (see **Figure 18-1**). Industries are required to keep Material Safety Data Sheets (MSDS) on all the potentially hazardous materials used, stored, or produced in the facility. A copy of the MSDS sheet is supposed to be sent with the patient to the hospital.

A placard posted on all four sides of the truck transporting hazardous materials is used to identify either the type or identification number of the hazardous materials being transported. The driver carries shipping papers that identify the hazardous materials onboard. Similar regulations govern railway, shipping, and airline transportation of hazardous materials as well.

Manufacturers of hazardous materials have 24-hour phone numbers available to answer questions regarding their products. Local fire departments and

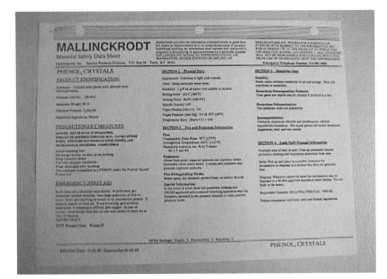

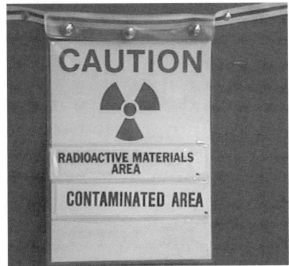

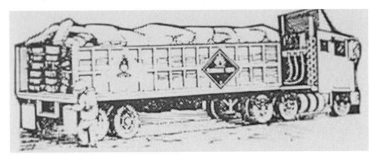

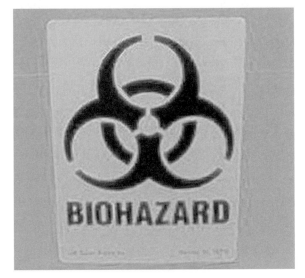

Figure 18-1 A MSDS Sheet, Two Biohazard Placards, and HAZMAT Truck

EMS agencies are also excellent resources for HAZMAT incidents in the community. Regional poison centers have a wealth of information available on the effects and treatment for many different substances and toxins.

Radiation Injury

Radiation occurs when an unstable atom emits either alpha or beta particles, or gamma rays. Neutron-type radiation injuries also may occur, but these are uncommon and are found only in high-technology situations, as with nuclear reactors. The first three types of radiation are discussed in **Table 18-1**.

Irradiation Versus Contamination

Radioactive materials may be in liquid, solid, or gaseous form. Contamination may be either external or internal.

External contamination occurs when there are radioactive alpha or beta particles on the patient or the patient's clothing. With external contamination, it is critical that the contamination be contained to prevent transmission to other areas on the patient or to caregivers.

Table 18-1   Types of Radiation

Type of Radiation	Characteristics	Safety Issues
Alpha	• Heavy particles that travel slowly and penetrate poorly • Stopped by paper or clothing and do not penetrate past the epidermis	• Cause internal contamination when ingested, inhaled, or absorbed through open skin
Beta	• 1/7,000th the size of alpha particles. • Penetrate into the dermal layer of the skin • Stopped by protective clothing	• May cause burns if left on the skin • Cause little damage unless internal contamination occurs
Gamma (Electromagnetic rays)	• 10,000 times more penetrating than alpha particles and 100 times more than beta particles • Stopped by lead shields	• Penetrate deep into tissues and cause damage to radiosensitive organs • Eyes are very sensitive to gamma rays. • Cataracts may appear.

Internal contamination is much more serious and occurs when the patient ingests, inhales, or absorbs radioactive particles. In these cases, the radioactive materials may be found in the cells, tissues, and organs, such as the liver, thyroid, kidney, and bone. Radiation continues to contaminate other tissues until the radioactive particles are removed or completely decay.

A patient is contaminated if there are radioactive particles on his or her body or clothing. The patient is a risk to caregivers because this contamination may spread. A special machine called a Geiger™ counter is used to detect radioactive particles on a patient during the decontamination process (see **Figure 18-2**).

Irradiation occurs when gamma radiation passes through or penetrates the body, similar to when an x-ray beam passes through the body. This patient is not a risk to others because no radioactive particles remain on the body. A radiation detector does not detect radioactivity from a patient who has been irradiated. However, it is possible that a patient may be a victim of both irradiation and contamination. Patients may exhibit delayed complications of exposure to radioactive materials, such as chromosomal changes, which may cause birth defects. Other serious long-range effects include sterility, anemia, and cancer.

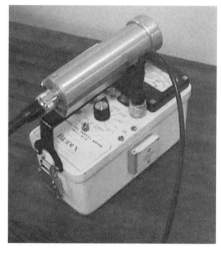

Figure 18-2   Geiger Counter
Courtesy of Mineralab, Prescott, AZ.

Prenotification

Before a patient with radioactive contamination arrives at the ED, the institution typically receives enough notice to establish a decontamination area. Note that the decontamination area is not always located in the ED. Sometimes the decontamination area is set up in the morgue because this area has good access to the outside and is usually somewhat separated from the main part of the hospital. Some institutions have special rooms separate but adjacent to the ED for the purpose of decontamination. Supplies for the decontamination area must be stored in that designated area. The nurse notifies additional personnel who are involved in one capacity or another with this type of situation.

Figure 18-3 A HAZMAT Area Roped Off

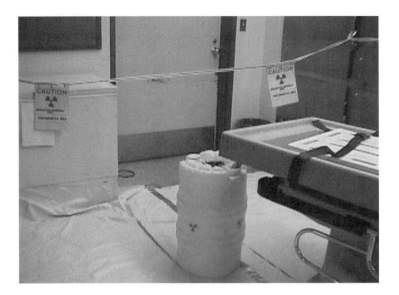

The ET may be asked to assist with the following procedures in preparation for the arrival of a patient contaminated by radiation.

- Cover pathways leading from the ambulance to the decontamination area with plastic, paper, or sheets. The area is roped off and a radioactive sign is attached until the area is cleared by the radiation safety officer (see **Figure 18-3**).

- Remove all nonessential equipment from the decontamination area or cover with plastic.

- Divide contaminated and clean areas of the room by placing 2 inch tape on the floor and at the entrance to the decontamination room.

- Obtain trash and linen containers for contaminated material.

- Women who are pregnant or have a chance of being pregnant should not be permitted anywhere near this area.

Preparation tips for the decontamination team:

- Use the restroom since the decontamination process may be lengthy.

- Attach a film badge with your name to outer clothes.

- Put on surgical scrubs, including (see **Figure 18-4**):
  - Waterproof shoe covers with pant legs taped to shoe covers
  - A surgical hood
  - A waterproof surgical gown
  - Surgical gloves taped to the cuffs of the gown
  - A second pair of gloves, not taped, so they are easy to change if they are torn or contaminated
  - Attach an outside dosimeter to the neck area so it is not easily contaminated

When the patient arrives to the ED, the hospital safety officer and a physician should meet the ambulance and examine the patient. Patients who are contaminated and in critical condition are taken straight to the decontamination area without taking the time to remove their clothing. Patients who are stable and contaminated are disrobed in the ambulance and then brought to the decontamination area. In either case, the patient is covered

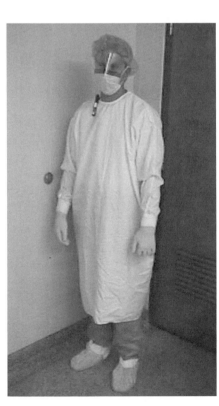

Figure 18-4 A Person Wearing a Gown and a Dosimeter

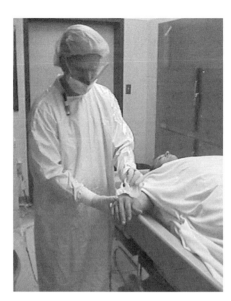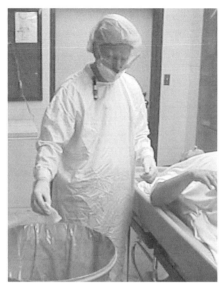

Figure 18-5 A HAZMAT Decontamination Table with a Person Being Decontaminated

with a sheet prior to being taken to the decontamination area. If the patient is not contaminated, he or she is brought to the ED.

Ambulance personnel remain with the ambulance until they and the ambulance have been monitored for contamination and decontaminated, if necessary.

Patient Evaluation and Treatment

As with all patients, airway, breathing, and circulation (ABCs) are assessed and any life-threatening problems are treated before continuing with the decontamination process (see **Figure 18-5**).

Decontamination Process

- Remove the patient's clothing if this has not already been done.
- The radiation safety officer assesses the patient, including the back.
- The location and amount of radiation is documented by the nurse.
- Obtain swabs of the nostrils, ears, mouth, and other contaminated areas and place the specimens in plastic bags and labeled for future analysis.
- Irrigate open wounds with normal saline solution for at least three minutes.
- Monitor for radiation with use of the Geiger™ counter and repeat irrigation, as needed.
- If contamination persists, consider surgical debridement of wounds; save and monitor all tissue removed.
- Rinse contaminated eyes with saline solution according to hospital policy.
- Rinse contaminated ear canals gently, suctioning frequently.
- To rinse the nostrils or mouth, turn the patient's head to the side or down and rinse gently, suctioning frequently to prevent fluid from entering the stomach.

- Insert a nasogastric tube is into the stomach to monitor contents. If contamination exists, the nurse lavages with water or normal saline solution until contents are clear of contamination.

- Medication may be given to interfere with absorption or speed the elimination of radiation from the gastrointestinal tract.

- Wash intact contaminated skin gently with soap and tepid water for three minutes, observe for any changes in condition, and repeat as necessary.

- Shampoo contaminated hair with mild soap for three minutes, monitor, and repeat if necessary. If contamination persists, hair may be clipped but not shaved.

- Collect all rinsed fluids in a special container; these fluids should not be allowed to enter the public sewer system.

Removal of a Patient from the Decontamination Room

- Dry the patient thoroughly.

- Reswab all previously contaminated areas if requested and label with the site and time and post decontamination. Swabs are given to the radiation safety officer for future analysis.

- The radiation safety officer monitors the patient and anything the patient comes in contact with.

- Place a new covering on the floor from the edge of the decontamination area to the door.

- Bring a clean stretcher into the room to the edge of the decontamination area.

- New personnel, who are not involved in the decontamination process, transfer the patient to the new stretcher.

- The radiation safety officer monitors the stretcher and wheels prior to the patient leaving the room.

Exit of the Decontamination Team

- Move to the line at the door and remove all protective clothing and equipment, placing it in a plastic bag marked "contamination."

- Remove outer gloves first, turning the gloves to the inside as they are removed.

- Give the dosimeter to the radiation safety officer.

- Remove tape at the ankles and wrists.

- Remove the surgical gown, turning it inside out and without shaking.

- Remove the scrub top.

- Remove the head cover.

- Remove the scrub pants.

- Remove one shoe cover, monitor the shoe, then step onto a clean area if the shoe is not contaminated.

- Remove the other shoe cover, monitor the shoe, then step completely over to a clean side if not contaminated.

- Remove inner gloves.
- Undergo total body radiologic survey by the radiation safety officer or designee.
- Shower and change into clean scrubs or uniform.

Chemical Contamination

Toxic chemicals are everywhere. Most work places have an assortment of potentially harmful chemicals, ranging from cleaning solutions, glues, and correction fluid, to copy machine fluids. There also are many harmful chemicals in homes, gardens, and garages. Examples include fertilizer, weed killer, fingernail polish remover, and common household cleaning products, such as cleanser, bleach, and metal polishes.

Decontamination Considerations

The method of decontamination for toxic chemicals may differ widely. Certain toxic chemicals must not be allowed to enter the public sewer system and must be collected and saved for disposal at a hazardous waste site. Some chemicals may emit dangerous gases and others may cause harm with skin contact.

Patients brought to the ED following exposure to a chemical toxin may have chemical burns, respiratory distress, or systemic effects from the toxin. They also may have associated trauma, or may be only contaminated with no apparent injury. Patients brought to the ED by EMS personnel usually have been partially, if not entirely, decontaminated prior to arrival. A more serious problem occurs if the patient arrives without warning from home or an industrial location and there has been no decontamination.

Not all patients who have been exposed to toxic chemicals are able to give that history on admission to the ED. In some cases, no one knows what kind of chemical was involved in the exposure. Prompt recognition of exposure and identification of the toxin are very important, not only for the patient but for the safety of the health care team. Clues that an exposure has occurred are listed below.

- Hazardous chemicals are manufactured, stored, or used at the site where the patient was found.
- Signage at the crash site identifies that chemicals were being transported by vehicles, such as trucks or railway cars.
- The patient reports irritation to the eyes, nose, or throat.
- A characteristic odor is present (i.e., the smell of almonds indicating cyanide poisoning).
- The patient or caregivers experience shortness of breath.
- Caregivers feel nauseated or dizzy when caring for the patient.

Substances such as carbon monoxide are odorless and tasteless and may not provide any sensory clues. Some chemicals have already reached toxic levels by the time any sensory clues are present, so treatment must not be delayed while waiting for evidence. If a contamination situation is not recognized early, the ED may be required to close for a period of time to be decontaminated, which is extremely costly and a loss of a valuable service to the community.

It is extremely important that the chemical be identified to be able to properly decontaminate the patient. Check for an MSDS because it identifies the chemical, describes its properties, and describes how to give first aid to victims of contamination. If the information on the MSDS is limited, look for a phone number to call for more information. If the exact name of the chemical is not available, it is at least helpful to know the type of chemical it is, such as corrosive, caustic, flammable, oxidizer, or another type.

The amount of harm a chemical causes depends on the concentration of the chemical and the length of time of the exposure. The decontamination process affects both of these factors. The concentration of the chemical is typically altered by dilution. If the decontamination occurs quickly, then the time the chemical is in contact with the body is reduced.

Decontamination procedures generally follow that of radiation decontamination, except that the floor covering must be a heavy-duty plastic, not paper or sheets. The ventilation system must be turned off in the decontamination room unless the room is vented to the outside. These measures protect the rest of the hospital from being contaminated by airborne particles.

Personal Protective Equipment

Protective equipment depends on the type of chemical exposure. This is why it is so important to know the name or type of chemical exposure. No one type of protective equipment is appropriate for use with every chemical. Information about specific protective equipment may be obtained through HAZMAT units from the fire department. Poison control centers, toxicologists on call at the hospital, or reference texts are other useful resources. Standard operating procedures for common chemical decontaminations also should be in place for quick reference.

If the chemical is harmful when inhaled, the ET staff needs respiratory protection other than a simple face mask, especially when the ventilation in the decontamination room has been turned off. HEPA respirator masks, such as those approved by the US Occupational Safety and Health Administration (OSHA) for tuberculosis protection, may be used to provide protection against some airborne chemical dust particles. Air purification devices that filter inhaled air are available but unfortunately they are generally designed to filter out only specific chemicals in a limited range of concentrations.

A self-contained breathing apparatus (SCBA) may be required in very toxic situations. The HAZMAT unit with the fire department may need to be called in for assistance in these cases. It is not realistic to think that the ED will have this equipment readily available.

The ET also needs protection from splashes during the decontamination process. Wearing chemical-resistant clothing, including gowns, gloves, boots, and face shields, is necessary. Thus, the ED must have a variety of protective equipment on hand in anticipation of commonly expected exposure situations. It is impossible to be prepared for every eventuality, and once again the HAZMAT unit may need to be called in for assistance.

Decontamination Process

The goal of decontamination is to limit patient exposure to the harmful chemical and to prevent secondary contamination of caregivers. The removal of contaminated clothing eliminates a large amount of contamination. Place clothing in a sealed plastic bag and set the bag aside for disposal with the rest of the hazardous waste.

Irrigation with copious amounts or water is helpful for most types of chemical decontamination. Avoid using hot water since vasodilation of the blood vessels may hasten absorption of the toxin through the skin. It is also usually helpful to add liquid laundry detergent to the wash water, especially if the chemical is fat-soluble or has a petroleum base. Cornmeal or a soft brush may help remove certain chemicals that are not easily washed away with a stream of soap and water. Avoid vigorous scrubbing and stiff brushes because abrasions increase the absorption of the chemical through broken skin. Occasionally, neutralizing agents may be recommended. Do not delay water irrigation while staff is searching for these other supplies.

The wash water may need to be collected and treated as hazardous waste. The water is collected in barrels that catch runoff from the decontamination stretcher. The drain system may be connected to a holding tank that is pumped out later by an agency that handles hazardous wastes. A conscious and alert patient may be able to shower in the decontamination room while standing in a small child's pool that collects the water.

The priority for decontamination is as follows:

- Contaminated wounds

- Eyes

- Mucous membranes

- Skin

- Hair (As with radiation contamination, clip the hair but do not shave if it is unable to be decontaminated to avoid causing any abrasions to the scalp)

Completing the Decontamination Process

Knowing when the decontamination is complete is not an exact science. If the patient is awake and alert, he or she is able to tell when the irritation or burning sensation goes away. The patient's skin may have a different feel to it once the chemicals have been removed. Monitoring the pH of the skin and eyes is also helpful.

Biological Contamination

Many types of bacteria, fungi, viruses and other types of agents used in residential or industrial areas or those naturally occurring in the environment may pose a threat to health. Some of these agents are contagious, while others affect only those who are exposed to them. Treatment and patient care issues will follow hospital protocols.

Summary

The ET must use extreme caution to avoid exposure while treating patients who are exposed to hazardous materials. Staff members who become ill while caring for a patient create more problems in the ED. Therefore, the ET must be familiar with the institution's policies and procedures for the treatment of victims contaminated with either chemicals or radioactive materials. The time for practice is before an incident occurs.

Bibliography

Borak, J. (1991). *Hazardous materials exposure.* Englewood Cliffs, NJ: Prentice-Hall.

Cox, R. D. (1994). Decontamination and management of hazardous materials exposure victims in the emergency department. *Annals of Emergency Medicine, 23*(4):761–770.

Kirk, M.A., Cisek, J., & Rose, S.R. (1994). Emergency department response to hazardous material incidents. *Emergency Medicine Clinics of Northern America, 12*(2):461–481.

REAC/TS (Radiation Emergency Assistance Center/Training Site). *Oak Ridge Institute for Science and Education.* Oak Ridge, TN. www.orau.gov/reacts/registry.htm

Sanders, M. (2000). *Mosby's paramedic textbook* (2nd ed.). St. Louis, MO: Mosby-Year Book.

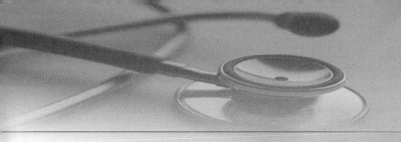

Glossary

Abdomen The body cavity that extends from the diaphragm to the pelvis; bounded anteriorly by the abdominal wall and posteriorly by the vertebral column. It contains the liver, stomach, intestines, spleen, kidneys, and associated tissues and vessels.

Amylase An enzyme produced by the body that helps to break down starch into simpler compounds.

Anemia A decrease of red blood cells or hemoglobin in the blood caused by a number of diseases and disorders.

Anterior Situated toward the front; opposite of posterior.

Antiemetic A medication that relieves vomiting.

Anus The opening of the rectum on the body surface.

Anxiety A vague, uneasy feeling or apprehension precipitated by new and unknown experiences.

Apnea The absence of spontaneous respirations.

Arrhythmia An irregular heartbeat.

Arthritis Inflammation of a joint.

Asepsis Absence of disease-producing microorganisms; being free from infection.

Assault A threat or attempt to make bodily contact with another person without that person's permission.

Asthma A disease of the bronchi of the lungs, whereby the individual has difficulty breathing, wheezing and poor air exchange.

Asystole A life-threatening cardiac condition characterized by the absence of electrical and mechanical activity in the heart; clinical signs include absent pulse and breathing.

Atrium A chamber or cavity, such as the right and left atria of the heart that send blood to the ventricles. Plural: atria.

Avulsion A soft-tissue wound in which the wound edges cannot be approximated; tearing away of a portion of the soft tissue; full-thickness loss of skin.

Battery An assault that is carried out.

Bloodborne Pathogens Pathogenic microorganisms present in human blood that can cause diseases in humans. These pathogens include, but are not limited to, hepatitis B virus, and human immunodeficiency virus (HIV).

Blood Pressure The pressure exerted by blood on the walls of the arteries, the veins, and the chambers of the heart.

Blunt Trauma Injuries that do not cause disruption of the skin.

Body Mechanics Efficient use of the body as a machine and as a means of locomotion.

Bradycardia Heart rate of less than 60 beats per minute.

Bradypnea Slow rate of breathing.

Cardiac Arrest A sudden and often unexpected stoppage of the heart beating resulting in death if resuscitative efforts such as CPR and defibrillation do not occur or are not successful.

Cardiac Output Volume of blood pumped from the left ventricle of the heart per minute.

Cardioversion The application of an electrical stimulant to the chest wall of a victim with an arrhythmia such as ventricular tachycardia with a pulse.

Catatonic A state of motor disturbances such as stupor or excessive activity and excitement, often seen in individuals with schizophrenia.

Catheter A tube for injecting or removing fluids.

Cervical Spine Stabilization (or Immobilization) Procedure to maintain alignment of cervical vertebra that consists of holding the head in a neutral position or application of a rigid cervical collar and placement of bilateral head support devices with tape.

Chyme Semifluid state that food is in when it leaves the stomach.

Closed Fracture A bone fracture that is not accompanied by a break in the skin.

Compartment Syndrome A potentially limb-threatening emergency resulting from increased pressure in a fascial (fibrous connective tissue) compartment from a variety of sources such as edema (swelling), bleeding or a cast; nerves and muscles are compressed as pressure rises inside the compartment. Often occurs with crush injuries and fractures.

Compliance The ability to adjust to pressure without damage to the organ.

Concussion Temporary loss of consciousness; no identifiable lesion.

Confidentiality The nondisclosure of privileged information.

Congenital Present at and existing from the time of birth.

Contraindicated When a treatment or intervention is not recommended for a specific condition and may cause serious harm if done.

Contusion An injury to soft tissues without breakage of skin; a bruise. Blood from the broken vessels accumulates in surrounding tissues, producing pain, swelling, and tenderness.

Coping Mechanisms Patterns of behavior used to neutralize, deny, or overcome anxiety. Factors that enable an individual to regain emotional balance after a stressful experience.

Core body temperature The temperature deep within a living body. The temperature obtained using a rectal thermometer will provide core body temperature.

Crisis A situation that develops when coping and defense mechanisms are no longer effective, resulting in high levels of anxiety, disorganized behavior, and the inability to function normally.

Crossmatching of Blood A process that analyzes the compatibility of two blood specimens.

Cyanosis A blue coloring of the skin and mucous membranes.

Defibrillation The delivery of an electric shock that is the definitive treatment for ventricular fibrillation or pulseless ventricular tachycardia.

Dermis The layer of skin just below the epidermis.

Diaphragm The muscle that separates the thorax from the abdominal cavity.

Displaced Fracture A bone fracture in which the proximal and distal sites are out of alignment.

Diverticula A pouch or sac formed by a protrusion of the mucous membrane through a defect in the intestine.

Documentation The written, legal record of all pertinent interventions with the patient including assessments, diagnoses, plans, interventions, and evaluations.

Do Not Resuscitate (DNR) An order specifying that there be no attempt to resuscitate a patient in the event of cardiopulmonary arrest.

Diastole The period of atrial or ventricular relaxation.

Diagnostic Peritoneal Lavage (DPL) A diagnostic procedure to detect blood or other contaminants in the abdominal cavity.

Distal Farthest from the point of reference, as from a center or the point of attachment or origin.

Distress Physical or mental anguish or suffering.

Doppler Ultrasound Flowmeter A device that uses sound waves to measure blood flow through veins and arteries, which transmits audible sounds reflecting the speed of the blood flow.

Dyspnea Difficult or labored breathing.

Dysrhythmia An abnormal cardiac rhythm; also known as arrhythmia.

Ecchymosis The collection of blood in subcutaneous tissues that causes a purplish discoloration.

Ectopic pregnancy Pregnancy outside the uterus; a life-threatening emergency.

Edema The accumulation of fluid in extracellular spaces.

Embolus A foreign body or air that circulates in the bloodstream until it becomes lodged in a vessel; plural: emboli.

Electrocardiogram (EKG, ECG) A graphic record that measures and records electric impulses of the heart.

Emphysema A disease of the lungs characterized by overinflation of the alveoli resulting in shortness of breath, difficulty breathing, and cyanosis.

Epidermis The superficial portion of the skin.

Epistaxis Nosebleed.

Esophageal Varices Enlargement of the veins in the esophagus; a sign of liver disease. Rupture of these veins can cause death.

Eupnea Normal respirations.

Eustress Normal, healthy form of stress.

Expiration The act of breathing out; exhalation.

Extension The straightening of a flexed limb.

Fat Embolus A mass (thrombus) of fat that can travel through the blood stream which can cause an obstruction in the blood vessels of the brain, kidneys, lungs and other organ systems resulting in death. Most often seen as a complication of long bone trauma, blunt trauma and/or orthopedic surgery.

Feces Intestinal waste products.

Fever Elevation of body temperature above normal; also known as pyrexia.

Fistula Any abnormal tube-like passage within body tissue. Some fistulas are created surgically; others occur as a result of injury or as congenital abnormalities.

Flaccid As seen in muscles that are weak, soft and flabby.

Flank The side of the body that extends from the ribs to the ischium.

Flexion The act of bending, or decreasing the angle at the joint between two bones.

Fluorescein Dye An orange-red dye used in solution which is applied to the eye to detect corneal injury.

Foley Catheter A urinary catheter that is placed in the bladder to continuously drain urine.

Fowler's Position Position with the head of the bed elevated and the hips and knees flexed.

Gag Reflex A reflex that occurs when the soft palate is stimulated often resulting in vomiting or "gagging."

Glaucoma A disease of the eye characterized by increased intraocular pressure that results in damage to the retina and the optic nerve which if left untreated can lead to blindness.

Glycosuria Glucose (or sugar) in the urine.

Greenstick Fracture A buckle or bend in a bone; fracture does not go through the entire bone.

Grief The physical, emotional, spiritual, cognitive, social, and behavioral response to loss.

Groin The area of the body where the thigh meets the abdomen.

Hematoma A tumor-like mass produced by coagulation of extravasated blood in a tissue or cavity.

Hemolysis The process of freeing a red blood cell of its hemoglobin by destruction of the cell membrane.

Hemoptysis Blood coughed up from the respiratory tract.

Hemothorax An injury resulting in blood accumulating in the pleural space.

Hepatitis Inflammation of the liver.

Herniate When one part of an organ or other body structure protrudes through a defect or natural opening into another muscle, membrane or bone.

Homeostasis A balanced state that the body maintains throughout various physiologic and psychological mechanisms as it responds to changes in the internal and external environments.

Hyperextend To extend a body part beyond its normal range of motion.

Hypertension Blood pressure elevated above the upper limit of normal (140/90 mm Hg).

Hyperthermia A greatly increased body temperature that results in heat cramps, heat syncope, heat exhaustion or heat stroke. A core body temperature of greater than 40°C (104°F).

Hypoglycemia Low level of glucose concentration in the blood.

Hypotension Blood pressure below the lower limit of normal (90/60 mm Hg).

Hypothalamus The part of the brain that coordinates the autonomic nervous system (ANS) which affects many involuntary actions in the body such as sweating, changes in arterial pressure and urinary output. It also affects sleep, alertness and reactions to pain and pleasure.

Hypothermia Body temperature below 35°C (95°F).

Hypoxia Decreased oxygen supply to the body tissues.

Immobilization Procedure that includes cervical stabilization as defined previously and the application of a backboard and straps.

Incontinent Lack of control of urinary functions.

Inspiration The drawing of air into the lungs.

Ischemia A decreased supply of oxygenated blood to a body organ or part.

Jaundice Yellow discoloration of the skin, mucous membranes, and the sclerae of the eyes.

Kilogram A unit of metric weight measurement (1 kg = 1,000 g or 2.2 lbs.).

Lateral Situated at the side.

Leukocyte A white blood cell; a component of the blood that protects the body against disease-carrying microorganisms.

Licensure The granting of permission by a competent authority to an organization or individual to engage in a practice or activity, such as nursing, after successfully meeting specific requirements.

Liter A metric measurement of volume (1 L = 1,000 ml or 1.1 qt).

Logroll Procedure in which the patient is turned as a unit; requires a team leader at the head of the patient who directs the turn and stabilizes the patient's head and cervical spine; other team members are positioned at the patient's side, usually one at the hips and one at the knees.

Mechanism of Injury Refers to the mechanism whereby the force or energy is transferred from the environment to the person; examples include motor vehicle crashes, gunshots, stabbings, burns.

Medial Situated toward the midline.

Medical Asepsis Practices designed to reduce the number and transfer of pathogens, also known as clean technique.

Mobility Ability to move, function.

Mottling Patchy discoloration of the skin related to peripheral vasoconstriction.

Nasopharyngeal The part of the pharynx above the soft palate.

Negligence Performing an act that a reasonably prudent person under similar circumstances would not do, or failing to perform an act that a reasonably prudent person under similar circumstances would do.

Neonate An infant from birth to 4 weeks of age.

Nonverbal Communication The exchange of information without the use of words; also known as body language.

Normal Sinus Rhythm A regular beat of the heart, with the rate in the adult of 60 to 100 beats per minute.

Nurse Practice Act A law established to regulate nursing practice.

Observation The conscious and deliberate use of the five senses to gather data.

Occult Blood Blood present in such minute quantities that it cannot be detected with the unassisted eye.

Open Fracture A fracture in which the broken end or ends of the bone have torn through the skin.

Ophthalmologist A physician who specializes in diagnosing and prescribing treatment for eye problems and is able to perform eye surgery.

Oropharyngeal The part of the pharynx behind the mouth and the tongue.

Pacemaker An electronic device that regulates the heart beat which may be implanted into an individual or applied temporarily to the outer wall of the chest.

Paradoxical Uneven motion, such as paradoxical rise and fall of the chest as seen in multiple rib fractures on one side of the chest.

Paresthesia An unusual sensation, such as numbness, tingling, or burning.

Parietal The outer wall of a cavity or organ.

Patent Open or not blocked, such as a patent airway.

Pathogen A disease-producing microorganism.

Personal Protective Equipment (PPE) Gloves, mask in combination with eye protection devices, gowns, aprons, surgical caps, and shoe covers worn as part of universal precautions as an infection control method.

Penetrating Trauma Injuries that cause penetration or disruption of the skin.

Perfusion The passage of fluid through a specific organ or area of the body.

Perineum The portion of the pelvic floor between the scrotum and rectum in the male and the rectum and vaginal orifice in the female.

Periorbital Around the eye socket.

Peristalsis Involuntary, progressive wave-like movement of the musculature of the gastrointestinal tract.

pH The symbol of hydrogen ion concentration. The pH range extends from 0 (pure acid) to 14 (pure base). pH of 7.0 indicates neutrality. A pH of less than 7.0 indicates acidity, a pH of greater than 7.0 indicates alkalinity.

Pharynx An area behind the nasal cavities that connects the mouth with the esophagus.

Plasma The liquid part of the blood.

Pleura The membranes covering the lungs and lining the inner aspect of the pleural cavity.

Pleural Cavity A potential space between the two pleural layers.

Pneumothorax An injury to the lung leading to accumulation of air in the pleural space with a subsequent loss of intrapleural pressure.

Posturing Abnormal movements made by patients who have a neurological defect.

Pressure Points Different locations on the body at which digital pressure may be applied to control bleeding.

Prone Lying face down.

Proximal Nearest to the point of reference.

Pulse A wave produced in the wall of an artery with each beat of the heart.

Pulse Oximetry A noninvasive technique that measures the oxygen saturation (SaO_2) of arterial blood.

Pyuria Pus in the urine.

Rape The sexual violation of a person by someone else who uses force, threats, and abuse.

Respiration The process of the exchange of oxygen and carbon dioxide within the body's tissues.

Respiratory Arrest A stoppage of breathing.

Respiratory Distress Difficulty breathing that if untreated will lead to respiratory arrest.

Restraint A device used to limit movement or immobilize a patient.

Retraction The act of drawing back, seen in the chest wall of a young child with respiratory distress.

Secretion A substance produced by the body such as sweat or hormones.

Serous Resembling blood serum; clear and watery in appearance.

Shock A syndrome resulting from inadequate perfusion of tissues and cells in the body leading to a decrease in the supply of oxygen and nutrients.

Sphygmomanometer An instrument used to measure arterial blood pressure.

Spinal Precautions The institution of cervical spine stabilization and/or immobilization using a cervical collar, backboard and/or manual stabilization.

Sterile Free from microorganisms.

Sternum A bony plate in the center of the chest that communicates with the cartilage of the ribs and clavicle. It consists of three parts: the manubrium, the body and xiphoid process.

Stool Excreted feces.

Strain Tissue damage or deformation that results from stress; dependent on the properties of the particular tissue involved.

Stress The relationship between a person and the environment that is appraised by the person as taxing or exceeding his or her resources and endangering his or her well-being.

Stressor The circumstances or event that creates the stress response.

Stroke Also known as a cerebral vascular accident (CVA), whereby there is a sudden rupture or blockage (thrombus) in a blood vessel in the brain.

Supine Facing upward, as in flat on the back.

Suture Also known as a stitch or stitches which close a wound.

Systole The contraction of the heart during which blood is forced into the aorta and pulmonary artery.

Tachycardia An abnormally fast heart beat; in an adult greater than 100 beats per minute.

Tachypnea Abnormally fast breathing.

Tendon A thick, white fibrous connective tissue that attaches muscles to bones.

Tension Pneumothorax A life-threatening injury to the lung that allows air to enter the pleural space on inspiration but cannot escape on expiration; rising intrathoracic pressure collapses the lung causing a mediastinal shift, compressing the heart and great vessels.

Tepid Lukewarm.

Testicular Torsion Twisting of the testicle or the spermatic cord occurring most commonly in children and adolescents. This is an emergency condition requiring surgical intervention.

Thrombus A blood clot attached to the interior wall of a vein or artery.

Trauma A Greek word meaning wound; used interchangeably with injury; damage to human tissue and/or organs resulting from the transfer of some form of energy from the environment to a human host; an injury that occurs when the energy is beyond the body's resilience.

Triage A process used to determine the urgency of need for emergency care based on assessment findings. The word triage means to sort or choose.

Tort A wrong committed by a person against another person or his property.

Tympanic Pertaining to the middle ear.

Universal Precautions An approach to infection control in which all human blood and certain human bodily fluids are treated as if known to be infected with HIV, hepatitis B virus, and other bloodborne pathogens.

Ventricle A small cavity or chamber; lower chambers of the heart.

Vital Signs Body temperature, pulse, respiratory rate, and blood pressure.

Wound An injury that results in a disruption in the normal continuity of a body structure.

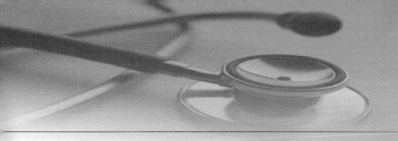

Common Medical Abbreviations

A & Ox3	alert and oriented to person, place and time
ā	before
ac	before meals
ABD	Abdomen
ABG	Arterial Blood Gases
ACLS	Advanced Cardiac Life Support
ADL	Activities of Daily Living
Adlib	as desired
AFib	atrial fibrillation
AIDS	Acquired Immunodeficiency Syndrome
am	morning
AMA	against medical advice
AMI	Acute myocardial infarction
ARD	Acute respiratory distress
asap	as soon as possible
ax	axillary
bid	twice a day
BC	blood culture
BLS or BCLS	Basic Cardiac Life Support
BM	bowel movement
BP	blood pressure
BR	Bed rest OR bathroom
BSA	body surface area
BVM	Bag-Valve-Mask
C & S	culture and sensitivity
c̄	with
cc	chief complaint
cc	cubic centimeters
CA	Cancer
CBC	complete blood count
CHF	Congestive Heart Failure
CNS	Central Nervous System
COPD	Chronic Obstructive Pulmonary Disease
CPR	cardiopulmonary resusitation
CSF	Cerebral spinal fluid
C-spine	cervical spine
CT	Computerized Axial Tomography
CVA	Cerebral Vascular Accident (Stroke)
CXR	Chest X-Ray

DKA	Diabetic Ketoacidosis
DM	Diabetes Mellitus
DNR	Do Not Resuscitate
DOB	Date of Birth
DTs	Delirium Tremens
D/C	discontinue
ECT	Emergency Care Technician
ED	Emergency Department
EKG or ECG	electrocardiogram
EMS	Emergency Medical Services
EMT-P	Emergency Medical Technician-Paramedic
EOC	End of Confinement—due date for pregnant woman
EOM	Extraoccular Movements
epi	Epinephrine
ET	endotracheal tube
ETA	Estimated Time of Arrival
ETOH	alcohol
FB	foreign body
FBS	fasting blood sugar
FOS	Full of stool
FUO	fever of unknown origin
fx	fracture
GC	gonorrhea
GCS	Glasgow Coma Scale
GI	Gastrointestinal
GSW	Gun shot wound
GU	Genitourinary
Hb	hemoglobin
Hct	hematocrit
HEENT	head, ears, eyes, nose and throat
HOB	head of bed
HR	heart rate
HTN	hypertension
Hx	History
H/A	headache
I & O	intake and output
IM	intramuscular
IO	intraosseous
IV	intravenous

JVD	jugular vein distention		**PCN**	Penicillin
kg	kilograms		**PE**	Pulmonary Embolism
KVO	keep vein open (as in IV rate)		**PEA**	pulseless electrical activity
L & D	Labor and Delivery		**PERRLA**	pupils equal, round, react to light and accommodation
Lac	Laceration		**PICU**	Pediatric Intensive Care Unit
LLE	Left lower extremity		**PMHx**	Prior Medical History
LLL	Left lower lobe (of lung)		**po**	by mouth
LLQ	Left lower quadrant		**POV**	private occupied vehicle
LMP	Last menstrual period		**pr**	in the rectum
LOC	level of consciousness		**PRBC**	packed red blood cells
LOS	length of stay		**prn**	as needed
LP	Lumbar puncture		**PVC**	Premature ventricular contraction
LPN	Licensed Practical Nurse		**q**	every
LR	lactated Ringer's solution		**qd**	every day
MD	Physician		**qid**	four times a day
mg	milligrams		**qod**	every other day
MI	Myocardial Infarction (heart attack)		**RBC**	red blood cell
ml	milliliters		**RN**	Registered Nurse
m/o	months old		**ROM**	Range of Motion
NA	Nursing Assistant		**RSI**	Rapid sequence intubation
NG	nasogastric tube		**Rx**	Prescription
NKA	No Known Allergies		**sl**	sub lingual
NP	Nurse Practitioner		**SOB**	Short of breath
npo	nothing by mouth (no food or drink)		**SQ**	subcutaneous
NRB	Non-rebreather mask		**stat**	immediately
NS	0.9% Normal Saline solution		**STD**	sexually transmitted disease
NSR	normal sinus rhythm		**SVT**	supraventricular tachycardia
NVD	Nausea, Vomiting, and Diarrhea		**Sx**	Symptoms
N/A	not applicable		**T & C**	type and cross
n/c	nasal cannula		**TB**	Tuberculosis
N/V	Nausea and vomiting		**TC**	throat culture
O₂	Oxygen		**TKO**	to keep open (same as KVO)
OD	right eye		**TIA**	Transient Ischemic Attack
O.D.	over dose		**tid**	three times a day
OG	orogastric		**Tx**	treatment
OJ	orange juice		**US**	ultrasound
OR	Operating Room		**VD**	venereal disease
OS	left eye		**VF**	ventricular fibrillation
ou	both eyes		**VT**	ventricular tachycardia
oz	ounce		**WBC**	White blood count
p̄	after		**WNL**	Within normal limits
PA	Physician Assistant		**wt**	weight
PACU	Post Anesthesia Care Unit		**x̄**	except
PALS	Pediatric Advanced Life Support		**XTL**	cross table lateral x-ray
PASG	pneumatic anti-shock garments (MAST trousers)		**y/o**	years old
pc	after meals			

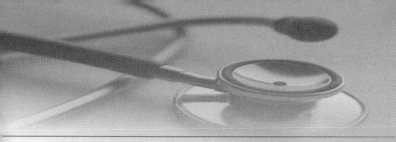

Index